# SURVIVE NOW
# THRIVE LATER

Cool Gus Publishing
http://coolgus.com

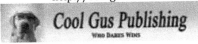

ISBN: 9781621253051

# SURVIVE NOW THRIVE LATER

## BOB MAYER

# Survival Triage priorities:

Breathing.
Bleeding.
Broken.

## BREATHING

### CHOKING—SELF HEIMLICH

1. Try to cough object up. If you cannot get it out, you must act quickly, before you lose consciousness.
2. Make a fist. Place it on your abdomen just above your navel and *below* your ribcage.
3. Hold the fist with your other hand for leverage.
4. Drive your fist in and up. Use a quick j-shaped motion. Repeat.
5. If the object does not dislodge, quickly find a stable object waist high, such as the back of a chair, a table, or a counter-top. With your hands still in place, bend over it, brace your hands. Drive your body against the object.
7. Repeat until the object dislodges.

### CHOKING—OTHER—HEIMLICH ADULT

1. From behind, wrap your arms around the victim's waist.
3. Make a fist and place the thumb side of your fist against the victim's upper abdomen, below the ribcage and above the navel.
4. Grasp your fist with your other hand and press into their upper abdomen with a quick upward thrust. Do not squeeze the ribcage; confine the force of the thrusts to your hands.
5. Repeat until the object has been expelled.

### CHOKING-OTHER-INFANT

1. Lay the child down, face up, on a firm surface.

2. Kneel or stand at the victim's feet, or hold the victim on your lap, facing away from you.

3. Place the middle and index fingers of both your hands below his rib cage and above navel.

4. Press in with a quick upward thrust. Do not squeeze the rib cage. Be gentle.

5. Repeat until object is expelled.

## NOT BREATHING—OTHER-CPR

1. Check the victim for responsiveness. If not responsive or not breathing or not breathing normally, call 911. Place the phone next to the victim and put in speaker mode. If necessary, the dispatcher can help you with instructions.

2. If the victim still is not breathing normally, coughing, or moving, begin chest compressions. Push down on the center of the chest 2 to 2.5 inches, 30 times. Pump hard and fast at a rate faster than one per second. After 30:

3. Tilt the head back and lift the chin. Pinch the nose and cover the mouth with yours. Blow until you see the chest rise. Do this 2 times. Each breath should take 1 second.

4. Go back to 30 compressions.

5. 2 breaths.

6. Continue until help arrives.

7. If doing two person CPR, the person compressing stops while the other person gives the 2 breaths.

## BLEEDING

**How to stop life-threatening bleeding. Signs of life-threatening are:**

Spurting blood.

Blood that won't stop.

Blood that is pooling on the ground.

Clothing that is soaked with blood.

Bandages that are soaked with blood.

Loss of all or part of a leg or arm.

Continued bleeding in a victim who is confused and unconscious.

**The key is to find and compress the bleeding blood vessel to stop the flow of blood.**

1. Find the source of the bleeding. Remove clothing from over the wound.

2. Apply pressure. Any cloth will do, but if you have the Quikclot you should have, that will help. 3. If the wound is deep, stuff the cloth/bandage into the wound.

4. Put a compression bandage on the wound, if available. Push down as hard as you can.

5. If a compression bandage is not available, apply continuous pressure until help arrives.

### Tourniquet

For life-threatening bleeding from an arm or leg and the above doesn't work.

1. Wrap the tourniquet around the limb 2 to 3 inches above the source of the blood. Do NOT put it on a joint. Go above the joint if necessary.

2. Pull the free end of the tourniquet as tight as possible and then secure it.

3. Twist the windlass until bleeding stops. Secure it in place or hold it.

4. Note the time it was applied.

### BROKEN

Unless BROKEN is a compound fracture with life-threatening bleeding, stabilize the patient, and look further in this book for how to treat.

# Table of Contents

INTRODCTION 11

FIRST AID 28

WATER PROCUREMENT 69

FOOD PROCUREMENT 83

BUILDING A SHELTER AND STARTING A FIRE 92

NAVIGATING, TRACKING 103

SPECIFIC ENVIRONMENTS AND EVENTS 112

STOCKPILE, SCAVENGE, SUSTAIN 146

CONGRATULATIONS 155

SUSTAIN AND THRIVE 156

THE KEY PHRASE TO REMEMBER: SURVIVAL 159

ABOUT BOB MAYER 171

NON FICTION BY BOB MAYER ERROR! BOOKMARK NOT DEFINED.

FICTION BY BOB MAYER ERROR! BOOKMARK NOT DEFINED.

COPYRIGHT ERROR! BOOKMARK NOT DEFINED.

# Introduction

*You Can Do It!*

*STAY CALM. THINK. TAKE CHARGE.*

## THE FIRST FIVE THINGS TO DO IN AN EMERGENCY

**FIRST**

Do a First Aid triage of yourself.
Assess the immediate situation.
If in immediate danger, get to a safe place.
What are the priorities of threats?

**SECOND**

Call for help

**THIRD**

Do a First Aid triage of others.

Breathing
Bleeding
Broken

Can the wounded be moved?
What is the status of your family/team? How will those not present assemble? IRP? ERP?

**FOURTH**

Assess the environment. Can you stay or do you need to leave?
If staying, check your supplies: water, communication, food and medical.

11

If leaving, dress in emergency clothing, take your Grab-n-Go bag.

If leaving, are you going to the ERP?

If leaving, and not going to Emergency Rally Point, what is your destination? Priorities being shelter, water, food, medication.

**FIFTH**

Once in a safe place, assess the overall situation and make long term plans.

More detail on each of these shortly.

This book is a quick reference guide for surviving emergencies and natural disasters.

This book assumes you have prepared to at least a mild emergency level using *Prepare Now-Survive Later*. That means you have a basic Grab-n-Go bag at home, in your car and at work/school, and your house has supplies at a baseline level. Your family/team has a designated Immediate Rally Point (IRP) and Emergency Rally Point (ERP).

You have conducted an Area Study & Emergency and Threat Analysis. You have prepared for the most likely threats in your area.

If you are using this book, you are currently in an emergency situation or one is imminent.

**The Five Key Elements of Survival**
Water
Food
First Aid
Shelter
Fire

**Develop a priority for survival based on the situation.**

There are five fundamentals to survival: water, food, first aid, shelter and fire. However, their priority will be different based on your situation. For example, in a cold weather, mountain environment, fire and shelter will be more important than in a temperate environment. If you are injured, then, of course, first aid would be a priority. Food is usually a last priority initially in a survival situation because we can go a lot longer without food than some of the other things, particularly water.

If your situation changes, you need to change your survival priorities. It should constantly be evaluated and updated.

## The Rule of Three
You can survive three minutes without air.
You can survive three hours without a regulated body temperature.
You can survive three days, depending on environment, without water.
You can survive three weeks without food.

This is why I put immediate action for lack of air before anything else in this book, even the Table of Contents. Thumb through this book, familiarize yourself with the way its laid out. Bookmark sections so you can find them easily.

**The book is structured as follows:**
First: FIRST AID
Second: WATER PROCUREMENT
Third: FOOD PROCUREMENT
Fourth: BUILDING SHELTER & STARTING A FIRE
Fifth: NAVIGATING, TRACKING
Sixth: SPECIFIC ENVIRONMENTS AND EVENTS

Seventh: STOCKPILE, SCAVENGE, SUSTAIN
Eighth: THRIVE LATER

## The First Five Things to Do in an Emergency.

Every situation is different and this is just a guideline. Always make sure your priority is safety for yourself first, then others. You can't help others if you don't take care of yourself.

### *First*:
Do a First Aid triage of yourself. Breathing. Bleeding. Broken.

Are you stabilized?

Can you move?

Assess the immediate situation. Take charge.

If in immediate danger, get to a safe place. If you're not in immediate danger, look around.

What are the priorities of threats? Other people will probably be panicking. Don't get caught up in that. Be aware that any situation can get worse. In fact, assume it will be. Also, having done your Area Study, you know there are after-effects of various emergencies and natural disaster. Earthquakes around the coast can lead to tsunamis. A terrorist attack could have a follow on attack for first responders. A hurricane can lead to broken gas lines which lead to a fire danger.

Check for smoke, gases and fumes. Locate and shut off the source if possible. Fires, earthquakes, bombs, etc. produce structural instability. Just because the roof is still there, doesn't mean it will stay there.

If in a car accident, turn off ignition, look out for pools of gas or any smoke.

### *Second*:
Call for help. Dial 911. Yell. Blow a whistle. Tap on a pipe with a piece of metal. Whatever is appropriate to the

event. If you're performing CPR, yell at someone nearby to call for help. Tell them what to say.

Getting trained personnel on the scene quickly is the best assistance you can render others. If you talk to a dispatcher, give a succinct summary of the situation: Location; what the emergency is; how many casualties and an estimate of condition; any potential threats.

If it is a mass casualty event, let them know that right away as the response will be different as a single responding unit would be overwhelmed.

### Third:

Do a First Aid Triage of others. Triage comes from the French word 'to sort'. The goal is to rapidly assess and prioritize a number of injured individuals and do the most good for the most people. The key here is it IS NOT to do the best for *every* individual.

First, make sure the injured are not in imminent danger.

How many are injured? How badly?

Who can assist you?

Can assistance get to you?

Your triage is what is at the beginning of the book: breathing and bleeding.

Professionals triage as follows:

| Triage | |
| --- | --- |
| Immediate (Red tag) | Victim will not survive without immediate care (example: not breathing, major hemorrhagic bleeding) |
| Delayed (Yellow tag) | Victim needs medical care within 2-4 hours (example, compound fracture, but not hemorrhagic bleeding) |
| Minimal (Green tag) | Stable and ambulatory, but may need some medical care. Get these people to help you. |
| Expectant (Black tag) | The victim is deceased or not expected to live (example, open fracture of cranium with brain damage; multiple penetrating chest wounds) |

Can the wounded by moved if they have to be? Do you have the means to move them?

If immediate help is on the way, don't take any unnecessary risks. Don't move an injured person unless they are in danger. Don't treat past life-saving measures. Let the professionals do their job when they arrive. Your job in this case, is to maintain until helps arrives.

What is the status of your family/team? If some members aren't present, where are they? Can you communicate with them and arrange to meet? If you can't communicate with them, can you contact your out of area emergency contact? If that's not possible the priority of meeting locations will be in order: home, IRP, ERP.

**Fourth**:

Assess the environment. Can you stay or do you need to leave? Do you have adequate shelter where you are for the environment? If you're staying, at home, at the IRP, ERP, work, school, wherever, inventory your supplies and gather what you can. Focus on water, communication, food and medical.

If leaving and can, dress in your emergency clothing. Take your Grab-n-Go bag (home, car or work/school). If leaving, are you going to IRP to meet family/team? Or is it best to go direct to the ERP?

If you're leaving and not going to any of those, what is your destination? Your out or area emergency contact? Are they clear of the emergency or disaster? The destination should be chosen by priority among shelter, water, food, and medication.

**Fifth**:

Once in a safe place, assess the overall situation and make long term plans.

## THE 3 PHASES OF SURVIVAL
## STOCKPILE, SCAVENGE, SUSTAINMENT

These are the three phases of emergency and catastrophe response and survival. They are based on two factors: level of emergency and length of the emergency.

### Three levels of Emergencies
Mild
Moderate
Extreme

*Mild*: You experience some discomfort from your normal routine for no more than 48 hours, but it is not life threatening. Example: Your power goes off for a day or two.

*Moderate*: You experience a large change from your normal routine, either natural or man-made, which is not immediately life threatening but has the potential to become so if not dealt with, and/or it continues. Example: Your power goes off for five days or more. Your car slides off the road in a remote area and you are trapped inside. A powerful hurricane is approaching. A 5.0 or greater earthquake strikes.

*Extreme*: A catastrophic natural or man-made event that immediately threatens your life and the lives of all around you, and if it continues, will be a constant threat. Example: A tsunami hits your coastal town. A tornado destroys your home. Nuclear, biological and chemical warfare/terrorist attack. A 7.0 or greater earthquake. The collapse of civilization. A pandemic with a high transmission and kill rate. Assume the worst until the situation stabilizes.

Length of emergency/catastrophe depends on how widespread it is, how severe, and how long it takes society to recover, if at all. There are too many variables to make any definitive answers.

Some extreme emergencies could be very short in duration. For example a severe car crash. A mild emergency that continues, might have a severe, long-term effect, such as a drought that doesn't abate. There could be a slow economic failure that will take years. Thus there are three phases to emergency and catastrophe survival that have no set time limits because the variables are so many and affect each other. These phases are:

### Three Phases of Survival
Stockpile
Scavenge
Sustainment

*Stockpile*: Initially, you will live off of your stockpile. This is what you have in your home, what you have in Grab-n-Go bags and what you have in your ERP. For those who are not prepared, their stockpile is poor or non-existent. It consists of what they might have on hand and what they are desperately trying to buy before a catastrophe; *if* there is warning.

*Scavenge*: This will occur both legally and illegally. After a disaster, people are desperate for supplies, particularly drinkable water. This is why in *Prepare Now-Survive Later*, there was a priority to what you needed to stockpile. Since power might well be out, cash will be the initial basis of barter. If cash loses its value (and cash is ultimately only valuable because we believe its valuable, it has no intrinsic value), then water, medicine, food, shelter, ammunition, etc. will become the currency of barter. That is while people are still willing to barter. Illegal scavenging is when people take what they want. Whether by gathering or by force.

*Sustainment*: This is when people will live off the land in a mixture of scavenging and hunting, gathering, farming and livestock. Some people are already living at a sustainment level. It's called living off the grid. However, unless those people are not only off the grid but unknown, in an extreme, long term emergency, they will become targets for illegal scavengers.

In your situation, because you have adequately stockpiled for at least a mild emergency, you will initially be in stockpile mode. Then you will probably resort to scavenging, while some will go to sustainment.

Thus the survival techniques in this book run the gamut from short-term emergencies where help is only cell-phone call away, to long term solutions.

I cover this more in detail in the Stockpile, Scavenge and Sustain portion of this manual.

### Should I Stay or Should I Go?

You've already considered the factors on when you should "bug out" from your home in *Prepare Now*.

However, there are so many possible emergency scenarios and catastrophes, that it's impossible for you to have covered all of them.

If an evacuation has been called, such as for a hurricane, you evacuate as soon as possible.

For some situations, smart people evacuate *before* the formal announcement. Wild fires are unpredictable and can move fast. Better to be safe than burned. The recent wild fires in Gatlinburg have claimed lives because they moved so much faster than expected.

There is a big difference between an evacuation and "bugging out".

An evacuation has the expectation that you would return to your home in the foreseeable future. In this case, it's as simple as driving away and checking into a hotel. However, if you live in an area where evacuations are likely, such as a hurricane zone, plan ahead. Have a location you know you can go to and get a room or people you can stay with.

First, let's discuss reasons *not* to bug out:

You have your primary stockpile of supplies in your house.

You have a community around you who knows you and you know (this could be a good thing or a bad thing).

There is no immediate or foreseeable threat to you and your home, whether natural or man-made.

When to bug out:

The most obvious time would be if the home is unlivable along with the IRP. This would happen in the case of an extreme emergency that affects the entire area. Ultimately the ERP will be the place for your team to meet up if all else fails.

However, making the decision to "bug out" is a very difficult one if your home is still livable. Because when you

20

bug out, there is a good probability you will not be returning to your home, so we're talking extreme emergency on a large scale where the ERP is your best option, rather than your evacuation point.

There are several predictors on deciding to go to the ERP.

Your home is no longer livable.

The emergency or disaster is something that is approaching you and can't be stopped. The primary example of this would be a pandemic.

The rule of law has completely broken down and now your home is a target and you cannot adequately defend it

Television stations go blank.

Local FM radio stations go off the air.

There are throngs of people trying to withdraw money from banks and ATMs in a panic.

Increased military presence, especially if its Federal forces, not National Guard. Federal military Army, Air Force and Marines can only be employed stateside in extreme emergencies. In your Area Study learn the difference and what National Guard units are nearby; what their unit patch is (on the left shoulder) and what unit designations would be marked on the bumpers of their military vehicles.

In cities, if garbage is piling up and not being picked up, eventually this will cause disease. It also indicates a slow breakdown of social order.

There is slim to no possibility of receiving aid. This latter is something people don't consider in mild or moderate emergencies. Localized emergencies always have the advantage of outside assistance coming in. If an emergency is on a national or international scale, this likelihood is drastically reduced.

A disturbing aspect of this is that while governments will call for evacuations, there really is no protocol for announcing things have gone to s$%t. In fact, it is unlikely that such a thing will ever be announced. The desire to avoid panic will often override reality. Thus you must make this decision on your own.

Make sure you can listen in on the Emergency Broadcast Stations with your crank radio. Also, a smart move is to monitor emergency transmissions in your area. Here is a free app that will allow you to do that. Often the emergency services are better informed than the general public. You can also get an idea of the scope of the emergency or disaster not only from what is being said, but the tone of the emergency personnel:

Scanner App: (Apple):
https://itunes.apple.com/us/app/scanner-radio-deluxe/id498405045?mt=8
Scanner App: (Android):

https://play.google.com/store/apps/details?id=com.scannerradio&hl=en

Some other factors to consider:

The power grid is down and isn't likely to come back up. Most urban areas can last about five days without power before society begins to unravel; often faster.

Water treatment and delivery systems have failed completely.

Long haul freight trucks are no longer moving. Most urban areas have enough food to last no more than a week.

You're running out of stocked supplies to the point where you're considering breaking into your main Grab-n-Go bag. Don't. Use it to get to your ERP.

Law and order has completely broken down.

### Survival Stress Factors

In 1967 Dr. Thomas Holmes and Dr. Richard Rahe developed the *Holmes Stress Scale*. They developed a stress point system for various life events. For example, the death of a spouse had a 100 point stress value. The holiday season had a 12 point stress value. You can go down the list and add up the events in your life and get the score. This is outside the survival situation.

*Consider an extreme survival situation well over 100.*

Then Holmes and Rahe predicted, based on your point total, the percentage chance that you have an illness or accident within the next two years. The higher the total, the higher the percentage.

Here are some of the most common, significant stressors:

Death—of someone close to you or even of strangers around you.

Moving—this is change in your life pattern. If you're evacuating, bugging out to your ERP, or to an safe location, you're moving.

Job Change—again, change and a degree of uncertainty. In an extreme emergency, you are changing jobs to becoming a survivalist.

Uncertainty—you don't know what is going to happen next.

Now, figure where a mild, moderate and extreme emergency would rank. Consider the fact that if you already have considerable stress in your life and you're high on the Holmes Scale, you might already be close to the breaking point.

Think about these stressors and the most common emotion they bring: fear. I don't think you can eliminate fear, nor would it be good to completely eliminate it, as there are times when fear serves a very useful purpose.

In an emergency situation, one issue is that there are many problems occurring at once. Often you will be overwhelmed. Your reaction will be the classic fight or flee. You will have a physiological response: your rate of breathing increases; your muscles will tense up; your body's stored fuel will be used at greater rates (carbohydrates and then fats); if you're bleeding, blood clotting increases; your senses become acute; your heart rate will increase, leading to a rise in blood pressure, in order to provide more fuel to your muscles. While this physiological reaction can help deal with the initial situation, it cannot be sustained for an extended period of time without adverse effects.

Understand that once that initial adrenaline rush and overall body response wear off, you will have a period of exhaustion. Be careful. Understand that exhaustion, hunger, wounds, etc. make you more susceptible to disease. It also clouds your judgment.

Stressors have a multiplying effect and you need to sort them out and deal with them individually before they overwhelm you. Here are some you will deal with in an emergency situation:

### Death, wounds, illness

You might well be surrounded by dead and dying people and also face the real possibility of your own mortality. The fact your death could come from multiple sources is also very hard to deal with. If you've been wounded or injured, this adds stress as it makes you consider the possibility that injury is mortal and also limits your ability to do the things needed to survive. Think of the last time you had the flu. Imagine being in a survival situation feeling like that. The reality is that illness has killed more soldiers over the course of history than battle. Over 600,000 men (lately revised to more likely 750,00) died in the Civil War, but two-thirds of those died from illness, not wounds.

### Guilt

Why me? Why was I spared? Was it luck? Fate?

While we can't help but ask these questions after an event that hurts or kills others and spares us, or destroys their property and not ours, they also can be used either positively or negatively. A negative response can lead us down the road of depression and despair. A positive response can be that whatever the reason, it is now your responsibility to value your life even more and try harder to survive.

### Uncertainty and lack of control

How do you deal with uncertainty? If you don't do well with it, start wrapping your brain around the fact that an emergency situation is full of uncertainty. Are you a control freak? Accept that you will have little control and little information in such a situation other than your immediate circumstances.

### Extreme environment

Later in this book I'll describe specific survival issues for extreme environments. One out of every six people who go up Mount Everest in an attempt to summit, die. Few people have ever experienced a night out in nature at 15,000 feet and minus 60 degrees. Or a desert at 120 degrees and a blasting sand storm. Ever wade chest deep through a swamp filled with snakes and alligators? All of those can be additional stressors.

### Hunger and thirst

What's the longest you've gone without eating? Do you know how much water you need to intake in your current climate every 24 hours to survive?

Being hungry and thirsty not only debilitates you physically, it stresses you because you will get more and more consumed with preserving and gathering water and food.

### Fatigue

People have literally fallen asleep into death. They become so tired and dispirited, that they curl up in a ball. There are situations where you simply cannot afford to fall asleep, such as when you are on guard duty for your team.

### *Isolation*

I focus on building a team, but the reality is that there's a good chance you will be alone in a survival situation, at least initially. How do you deal with being alone? Think of Tom Hanks in the movie *Cast Away*. Even though he was surviving on that island, ultimately the loneliness drove him to put his life at risk and go out to sea.

This factor is a big reason why I'm a fan of putting together a team and having a way for that team to link-up after a disaster happens, if they aren't together while it occurs. We'll discuss emergency rally points and link ups later.

THE KEY is that if you've done the basic preparation in *Prepare Now-Survive Later*, you are ahead of over ninety-five percent of other people facing the same emergency!

*I'm a big believer a few things done well are better than a lot of things done poorly or not remembered.*

*I focus on key items in each area. Entire books have been written about subjects such as emergency first aid, hunting, fishing, trapping, etc. If you want more on those topics, take a course, go out and practice, get specific guides. As you will see under Scavenge, knowledge and expertise are high on the list in terms of books and personnel.*

*I do not believe this is the only manual you should have for survival. But it is an excellent base from which to expand your base skills. For example, in hunting and trapping, I give you the most effective trapping technique using the snares you have in Grab-n-Go bag. Also you can improvise those snares. I don't go into all the field-expedient traps you can build because many are simply too time and energy consuming and difficult to do; but also, you're prepared for a more effective way. The same for shelters. I tell you how to build a field expedient shelter in various environments, but not the entire possible array.*

*My focus is to give a handful of the most effective tools for you to deal with emergencies and catastrophes.*

Take a deep breath. Check out the key word SURVIVAL at the end of this book to remind yourself what means. You've already done S: Sized up the situation, your surrounding, yourself and your equipment. Now remember, U: Use all your senses and Undue haste makes waste.

# FIRST AID

(Disclaimer: This is advice. But every situation
is different.
I am not a medical expert. I am passing on what I have
learned and what I've gathered from those who are.
Get professional medical assistance.)

### Survival Triage priorities:
Breathing.
Bleeding.
Broken.

### Lifesaving Steps
Remain calm and do not panic. Check yourself first,
then render aid to others.

Perform a rapid physical exam. Look for the cause of
the injury and follow the ABCs of first aid, starting with the
airway and breathing, but be discerning. A person may die
from arterial bleeding more quickly than from an airway
obstruction in some cases.

If you have your cell phone and power, you've already
downloaded Apps which can quickly guide you to First Aid
topics and even show you video of what to do along with
audio instructions. Use these Apps if you can rather than
trying to read instructions.

Here they are again.

## First Aid Apps

Red Cross First Aid (Apple)
https://itunes.apple.com/us/app/first-aid-by-american-red/id529160691?mt=8
Red Cross First Aid (Android)
https://play.google.com/store/apps/details?id=com.cube.arc.fa&hl=en
iTriage (Apple)
https://itunes.apple.com/us/app/itriage-symptom-checker/id304696939
iTriage (Android)
https://play.google.com/store/apps/details?id=com.healthagen.iTriage
CPR and Choking (Apple)
https://itunes.apple.com/app/cpr-choking/id314907949
CPR and Choking (Android)
https://play.google.com/store/apps/details?id=org.learncpr.videoapp


The information below is only for emergencies when no other option is available and is not the definitive word on First Aid.

# First Aid Topics Covered in Order

| | |
|---|---|
| Breathing | Health causes |
| | Emergency causes |
| | Symptoms |
| | Treatment—Heimlich/CPR |
| | Treatment--Allergic Reaction/Collapsed Lung |
| Bleeding | Symptoms of life-threatening bleeding |
| | Treatment of life-threatening bleeding |
| | Controlling bleeding—Pressure & Tourniquet |
| | Treating Open Wounds |
| | Burns |
| | Shock |
| Broken (Bone & Joints) | Fracture (closed and open) |
| | Dislocations |
| | Sprains |
| Water | Dehydration |
| | Heat Stroke |
| Food | Basics. Plant and Animal |
| Cold Weather Injuries | Frostbite and Hypothermia |
| Bites and Stings | Ticks, bees, wasps, spiders, scorpions, snakes |
| Personal Hygiene | |

## BREATHING

Since we can only survive three minutes without oxygen, breathing is a priority. At the beginning of the book I gave the Heimlich and CPR, but there are an array of breathing problems from a variety of source. I'll go over both again, but first, let's look at an array of possible problems:

Shortness of breath.

Unable to take a deep breath and gasping for air.

Feeling like you can't get enough air.

Not breathing.

### *Health Causes of breathing problems:*

Difficulty breathing is always a medical emergency.

Anemia (low red blood cell count)

Asthma

Chronic obstructive pulmonary disease (COPD), more commonly called emphysema or chronic bronchitis.

Heart disease or failure.

Lung cancer, or cancer that has spread to the lungs.

Respiratory infections, including pneumonia, acute bronchitis, whooping cough, croup and others.

Pericardial effusion (fluid surrounding the heart, including blood, that won't allow it to fill properly).

Pleural effusion (fluid surround the lungs, including blood, that compresses them).

### *Emergency Causes of breathing problems:*

Being at high altitude.

Blood clot in lungs.

Pneumothorax (collapsed lung).

Heart attack.

Injury to the neck, chest wall, or lungs.

Foreign matter in mouth of throat that obstructs the opening to the trachea.

Inflammation and swelling of mouth and throat caused by inhaling smoke, flames, and irritating vapors or by an allergic reaction.

"Kink" in the throat (caused by the neck bent forward so that the chin rests upon the chest) may block the passage of air.

31

Tongue blocks passage of air to the lungs upon unconsciousness. When an individual is unconscious, the muscles of the lower jaw and tongue relax as the neck drops forward, causing the lower jaw to sag and the tongue to drop back and block the passage of air.

Life-threatening allergic reaction.

Near drowning, with fluid build up in the lungs.

### *Symptoms*:
Rapid breathing.

Unable to breathe lying down and needing to sit up to breathe.

Very anxious or agitated.

Sleepy or confused.

Dizziness.

Cough.

Nausea.

Vomiting.

Bluish lips, fingers and fingernails.

Chest moving in an unusual way.

Gurgling, wheezing or whistling sounds.

Difficulty speaking or muffled voice.

Coughing up blood.

Rapid or irregular heartbeat.

If an allergy is causing the problem, there might be a rash or swelling of the face, tongue, or throat.

If an injury is causing the problem, there might be bleeding or a visible wound.

### *Treatment*:
*A key to remember is that leaning the head back opens the airway in the throat as much as possible.*

You can open an airway and maintain it by using the following steps.

*Step 1.* Check if the victim has a partial or complete airway obstruction. If he can cough or speak, allow him to clear the obstruction naturally. Stand by, reassure the victim, and be ready to clear his airway and perform mouth-to-mouth resuscitation should he become unconscious. If his airway is completely obstructed, administer the Heimlich until the obstruction is cleared.

*Step 2.* Using a finger, quickly sweep the victim's mouth clear of any foreign objects, broken teeth, dentures, sand.

*Step 3.* Using the jaw thrust method, grasp the angles of the victim's lower jaw and lift with both hands, one on each side, moving the jaw forward. For stability, rest your elbows on the surface on which the victim is lying. If his lips are closed, gently open the lower lip with your thumb. *Lean the head back to further open the airway.*

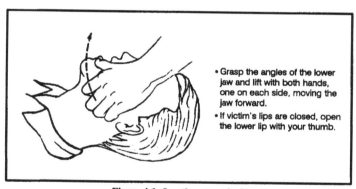

• Grasp the angles of the lower jaw and lift with both hands, one on each side, moving the jaw forward.
• If victim's lips are closed, open the lower lip with your thumb.

**Figure 4-1. Jaw thrust method.**

*Step 4.* With the victim's airway open, pinch his nose closed with your thumb and forefinger and blow two complete breaths into his lungs. Allow the lungs to deflate after the second inflation and perform the following:

*Look* for his chest to rise and fall.

*Listen* for escaping air during exhalation. *Feel* for flow of air on your cheek.

*Step 5.* If the forced breaths do not stimulate spontaneous breathing, maintain the victim's breathing by performing mouth-to-mouth resuscitation.

*Step 6.* There is danger of the victim vomiting during mouth-to-mouth resuscitation. Check the victim's mouth periodically for vomit and clear as needed.

Note: Cardiopulmonary resuscitation (CPR) may be necessary after cleaning the airway, but only after major bleeding is under control.

### SELF HEIMLICH

Try to cough object up. If you cannot get it out, you must act quickly, before you lose consciousness.

Make a fist. Place it on your abdomen just above your navel and *below* your ribcage.

Hold the fist with your other hand for leverage.

Drive your fist in and up. Use a quick j-shaped motion. Repeat.

If the object does not dislodge, quickly find a stable object waist high, such as the back of a chair, a table, or a counter-top. With your hands still in place, bend over it, brace your hands. Drive your body against the object.

Repeat until the object dislodges.

### CHOKING—OTHER—HEIMLICH ADULT

From behind, wrap your arms around the victim's waist.

Make a fist and place the thumb side of your fist against the victim's upper abdomen, below the ribcage and above the navel.

Grasp your fist with your other hand and press into their upper abdomen with a quick upward thrust. Do not squeeze the ribcage; confine the force of the thrusts to your hands.

Repeat until the object has been expelled.

## CHOKING--INFANT

Lay the child down, face up, on a firm surface.

Kneel or stand at the victim's feet, or hold the victim on your lap, facing away from you.

Place the middle and index fingers of both your hands below his rib cage and above navel.

Press in with a quick upward thrust. Do not squeeze the rib cage. Be gentle.

Repeat until object is expelled.

## PERFORMING CPR:

Check the victim for responsiveness. If not responsive or not breathing or not breathing normally, call 911. Place the phone next to the victim and put in speaker mode. If necessary, in most places, the dispatcher can help you with instructions.

If the victim still is not breathing normally, coughing, or moving, begin chest compressions. Push down on the center of the chest 2 to 2.5 inches, 30 times. Pump hard and fast at the rate faster than one per second. After 30:

Tilt the head back and lift the chin. Pinch the nose and cover the mouth with yours. Blow until you see the chest rise. Do this 2 times. Each breath should take 1 second.

Go back to 30 compressions.

2 breaths.

Continue until help arrives.

If doing two person CPR, the person compressing stops while the other person gives the 2 breaths.

### *Treatment Allergic Reaction/Collapsed Lung:*

*Dealing with a Severe Allergic Reaction leading to Anaphylaxis*:

Call 911 immediately.

See if they have epinephrine auto injector and use as the instructions on it indicate.

Keep them calm.

Have them lie on their back.

Raise their feet 12 inches and cover with a blanket.

Turn them on their side if they are vomiting or bleeding.

Make sure their clothing is loose.

*Dealing with a Collapsed Lung:*

A collapsed lung can be caused several ways including:

A puncture from a broken rib.

A puncture wound through the chest wall (a sucking chest wound).

A weak part of the lung that starts leaking.

*Signs and symptoms:*

Sudden pain on the affected side.

Shortness of breath.

Obvious wound to the chest.

If you have a stethoscope you can listen on that side of the chest and breath sounds are either absent or greatly decreased.

*Treatment*:

If it's a puncture wound and the object is still in place, leave it in place and call for help or get assistance.

If it's an open sucking chest wound allowing air in to the lung, bandage the wound, using an airproof material or bandage first, such as plastic wrap, a plastic bag, or gauze pads covered with petroleum jelly, sealing it, except for one corner, allowing air to escape, but not go in.

Do not:

Give the person food or drink.

Move the person unless absolutely necessary.

Place anything under their head to raise it as this will restrict the air passage.

Wait to see if their condition improves before getting help.

# BLEEDING

An average adult weighing between 150 and 180 pounds, has about 4.7 to 5.5 liters, or 1.2 to 1.5 gallons (5 to 6 quarts) of blood.

Losing 1 liter, or 1 quart, of blood will begin to send someone into shock. Losing 2 liters, 2 quarts, will induce severe shock. Losing 3 liters, 3 quarts, usually results in death.

### *Symptoms of life-threatening bleeding are*:
Spurting blood.
Blood that won't stop.
Blood that is pooling on the ground.
Clothing that is soaked with blood.
Bandages that are soaked with blood.
Loss of all or part of a leg or arm.
Continued bleeding in a victim who is confused and unconscious.

### *Treatment of life-threatening bleeding:*
**The key is to find and compress the bleeding blood vessel to stop the flow of blood.**

Find the source of the bleeding. Remove clothing from over the wound.

Apply pressure. Any cloth will do, but if you have the Quikclot you should have, that will help. If the wound is deep, stuff the cloth/bandage into the wound.

Put a compression bandage on the wound, if available. Push down as hard as you can.

If a compression bandage is not available, apply continuous pressure until help arrives.

## Tourniquet

For life-threatening bleeding from an arm or leg and the above doesn't work.

Wrap the tourniquet around the limb 2 to 3 inches above the source of the blood. Do NOT put it on a joint. Go above the joint if necessary.

Pull the free end of the tourniquet as tight as possible and then secure it.

Twist the windlass until bleeding stops. Secure it in place or hold it.

Note the time it was applied.

More details on all of these follow.

### *Controlling Bleeding:*

In a survival situation, you must control serious bleeding immediately because replacement fluids (IVs) are usually not available and the victim can die within a matter of minutes. External bleeding falls into the following classifications:

*Arterial.* Blood vessels called arteries carry blood away from the heart and through the body. A cut artery issues *bright red* blood from the wound in *distinct spurts* or pulses that correspond to the rhythm of the heartbeat. Because the blood in the arteries is under high pressure, an individual can lose a large volume of blood in a short period when damage to an artery of significant size occurs. Therefore, arterial bleeding is the most serious type of bleeding. If not controlled promptly, it can be fatal. *This is where you break the rule of three in the B—breathing, bleeding, broken—and bleeding is the number on priority.*

*Venous.* Venous blood is blood that is returning to the heart through blood vessels called veins. A steady flow of *dark red, maroon, or bluish* blood characterizes bleeding from a vein. You can usually control venous bleeding more easily than arterial bleeding.

*Capillary.* The capillaries are the extremely small vessels that connect the arteries with the veins. Capillary bleeding most commonly occurs in minor cuts and scrapes. This type of bleeding is not difficult to control.

You can control external bleeding by direct pressure, indirect (pressure points) pressure, elevation, digital ligation, or tourniquet.

**Direct Pressure**

The most effective way to control external bleeding is by applying pressure directly over the wound. This pressure must not only be firm enough to stop the bleeding, but it must also be maintained long enough to allow the bleeding to stop on its own.

Using a Quikclot bandage can help greatly.

If bleeding continues after having applied direct pressure for 30 minutes, apply a pressure dressing. This dressing consists of a thick dressing of gauze, a Quikclot sponge, or other suitable material applied directly over the wound and held in place with a tightly wrapped bandage or if need be, tape. It should be tighter than an ordinary compression bandage but not so tight that it impairs circulation to the rest of the limb if on an appendage. Once you apply the dressing, *do not remove it,* even when the dressing becomes blood soaked. If blood continues to come through, though, then you have a more serious problem. If bleeding stops, leave the pressure dressing in place for at least a day, after which you can carefully remove it and replace it with a smaller dressing.

In the long-term emergency, change bandages every day and inspect for signs of infection.

Signs a wound is infected: Expanding redness around the wound, including red streaks. Running a fever. Fluid draining that is cloudy or yellow/green pus or the wound is foul-smelling. Increasing tenderness, swelling or pain around the wound.

**Elevation**

Raising an injured extremity as high as possible above the level of the heart slows blood loss by aiding the return of blood to the heart and lowering the blood pressure at the wound. However, elevation alone *will not* control bleeding entirely; you must also apply direct pressure over the wound. If treating a snakebite, however, keep the extremity lower than the heart.

### Tourniquet

Use a tourniquet on a limb only when direct pressure over the bleeding point and all other methods did not control the bleeding. If you leave a tourniquet in place too long, the damage to the tissues can progress to gangrene, with a loss of the limb later. An improperly applied tourniquet can also cause permanent damage to nerves and other tissues at the site of the constriction.

What can you use for a field expedient tourniquet? Use something that is at least 1 inch wide out to 2 inches. Using something like parachute cord or string, that is too narrow, can cut into the skin. A pressure cuff can loosen. Using something too wide will make it too hard to tighten down. A belt is good. There are commercially available tourniquets, such as a CAT (Combat Application Tourniquet-- http://amzn.to/2gZEkF4 available for less than $20 at Amazon).

If you must use a tourniquet, place it around the extremity, between the wound and the heart, 2 to 4 inches above the wound site. Never place it directly over the wound or a fracture or a joint. Use a stick as a handle to tighten the tourniquet and tighten it only enough to stop blood flow. When you have tightened the tourniquet, securely bind the free end of the stick to the limb to prevent unwinding.

After you secure the tourniquet, clean and bandage the wound.

If you've applied this to yourself and you are alone, do not remove or release. You could loose too much blood in the process and pass out, then bleed out. In a buddy system, however, the buddy can release the tourniquet pressure every 10 to 15 minutes for 1 or 2 minutes to let blood flow to the rest of the extremity to prevent limb loss.

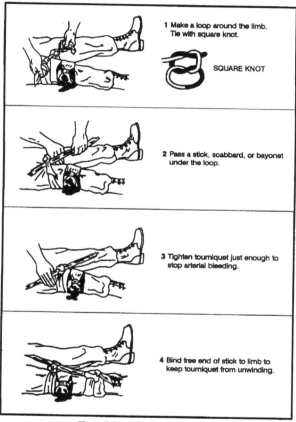

1 Make a loop around the limb. Tie with square knot.

SQUARE KNOT

2 Pass a stick, scabbard, or bayonet under the loop.

3 Tighten tourniquet just enough to stop arterial bleeding.

4 Bind free end of stick to limb to keep tourniquet from unwinding.

Figure 4-4. Application of tourniquet.

### Dangers of using a tourniquet:

Applying too loosely. This can cause bleeding to worsen as the venous (return) blood is blocked because it is under less pressure, but arterial blood still bleeds out.

Releasing it too soon, causing severe bleeding to resume. Also, this could cause venous blood to damage compressed blood vessels.

Leaving it on too long, causing neurovascular damage and tissue death. Permanent nerve, muscle and blood vessel damage occurs after about two hours. If the choice is between this and bleeding out, then go with keeping alive.

Periodic loosening could lead to the victim bleeding out. This is a damned if you do, damned if you don't scenario.

Applying a tourniquet to a victim with low blood pressure who is in shock or receiving CPR. If the person is revived, their bleeding will increase as blood pressure increases.

**Open Wounds**

If the bleeding has stopped, you must now treat an open wound. Beyond the problem of the tissue damage and blood loss, there is the great concern of infection. In a high moderate to extreme emergency, the lack of access to medical care makes infections a life-threatening situation. Better to prevent them, than have to deal with them.

Infection comes from dirt on the object that made the wound, on the individual's skin and clothing, or on other foreign material or dirt that touches the wound.

By taking proper care of the wound you can reduce further contamination and promote healing.

Clean the wound as soon as possible after it occurs by:
Removing or cutting clothing away from the wound.
Always looking for an exit wound if a sharp object, gun shot, or projectile caused a wound.
Thoroughly cleaning the skin around the wound.

Rinsing (not scrubbing) the wound with large amounts of water under pressure. You can use fresh urine if water is not available. Fresh urine is sterile.

The "open treatment" method is the safest way to manage wounds in survival situations. Do not try to close the wound by suturing or similar procedures. Leave the wound open to allow the drainage of any pus resulting from infection. As long as the wound can drain, it generally will not become life-threatening, regardless of how unpleasant it looks or smells.

Cover the wound with a clean dressing. Place a bandage on the dressing to hold it in place. Change the dressing daily to check for infection.

If a wound is gaping, you can bring the edges together with adhesive tape cut in the form of a "butterfly" or "dumbbell" bandage.

*To treat an infected wound*:

Place a warm, moist compress directly on the infected wound. Change the compress when it cools, keeping a warm compress on the wound for a total of 30 minutes. Apply the compresses three or four times daily.

Drain the wound. Open and gently probe the infected wound with a sterile instrument.

Dress and bandage the wound. Drink a lot of water.

Continue this treatment daily until all signs of infection have disappeared.

If you do not have antibiotics and the wound has become severely infected, does not heal, and ordinary debridement is impossible, consider maggot therapy, despite its hazards:

Expose the wound to flies for one day and then cover it.

Check daily for maggots. Once maggots develop, keep the wound covered but check daily. Remove all maggots when they have cleaned out all dead tissue and before they start on healthy tissue. Increased pain and bright red blood in the wound indicate that the maggots have reached healthy tissue. Flush the wound repeatedly with sterile water to remove the maggots. Check the wound every four hours for several days to ensure all maggots have been removed. Bandage the wound and treat it as any other wound. It should heal normally.

### Burns

Put out the fire. If clothes are on fire, remove, douse with water or sand, or roll on the ground until it is out. Remove charred clothing.

Immerse the burn in cold water for approximately 30 minutes if help isn't on the way.

Minor burns can be cooled using tap water.

Do NOT use ice or apply ice to the burn wound.

For burns caused by white phosphorous, pick out the white phosphorous with tweezers; do not douse with water.

Soak dressings or clean rags for 10 minutes in a boiling tannic acid solution (obtained from tea, inner bark of hardwood trees, or acorns boiled in water).

Cool the dressings or clean rags and apply over burns. Rest as an open wound.

Replace fluid loss.

Maintain airway.

Treat for shock.

### Shock

Shock is a life-threatening medical condition resulting from an insufficient flow of blood throughout the body. It can lead to other conditions such as lack of oxygen in the body's tissues (hypoxia), heart attack, or organ damage. If not treated, it can kill. Once shock sets in, unless treated, it will get worse quickly.

In an emergency situation, without immediate aid, people with survivable wounds and injuries will die from shock.

It's beyond the scope of this book, but having a trained person on your team who can administer IVs is a great boon. In Special Forces we trained on giving each other and even ourselves IVs.

Symptoms of shock:

Cold, clammy skin.

Pale, ashen skin.

Confusion and lack of alertness.

Rapid pulse.

Nausea or vomiting.

Enlarged pupils.

Weakness or fatigure.

Loss of consciousness.

### Prevent and Treat Shock

Assume anyone who is wounded or injured will go into shock, so treat everyone for it, regardless of whether symptoms appear.

If the victim is conscious, place on a level surface with the legs and feet elevated slightly.

If the victim is unconscious, place him on his side or abdomen with his head turned to one side to prevent choking on vomit, blood, or other fluids.

Once the victim is in a shock position, do not move him.

Maintain body heat by using blankets, coats, whatever is at hand.

If the person is wet, remove the wet clothing as soon as possible and replace with dry.

If conscious, and other wounds do not preclude, slowly administer small doses of a warm salt or sugar solution. If unconscious or there is an abdominal wound, do not.

Have them rest for at least a day to recover.

If its you, and you are alone, get to a shelter, rest, with feet slightly elevated.

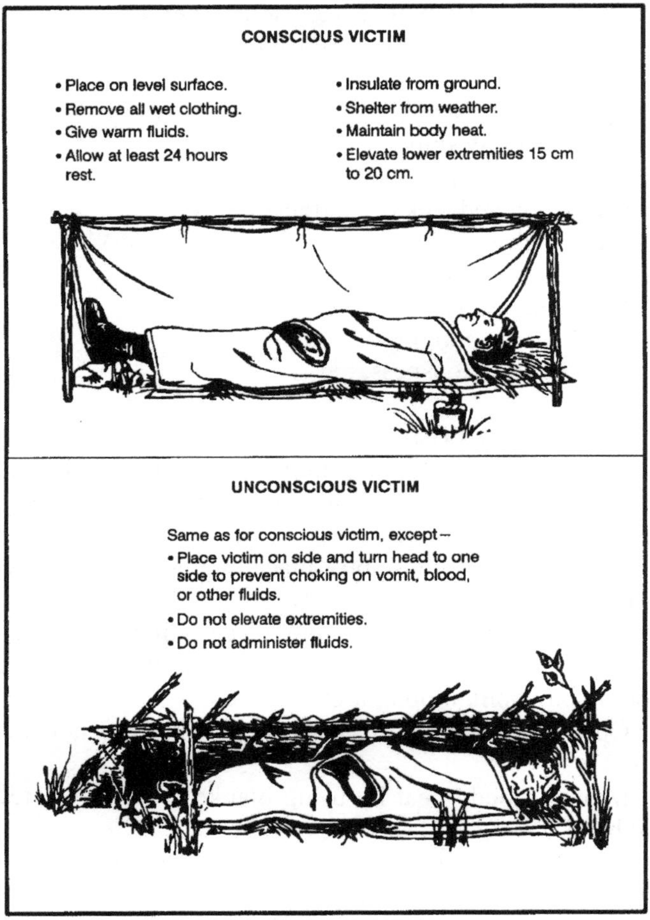

**CONSCIOUS VICTIM**

- Place on level surface.
- Remove all wet clothing.
- Give warm fluids.
- Allow at least 24 hours rest.

- Insulate from ground.
- Shelter from weather.
- Maintain body heat.
- Elevate lower extremities 15 cm to 20 cm.

**UNCONSCIOUS VICTIM**

Same as for conscious victim, except—
- Place victim on side and turn head to one side to prevent choking on vomit, blood, or other fluids.
- Do not elevate extremities.
- Do not administer fluids.

Figure 4-5. Treatment for shock.

# BROKEN—Bone & Joint Injuries

Bone and joint injuries include fractures, dislocations, and sprains.

**Fractures**

There are two types of fractures: open and closed. With an open (or compound) fracture, the bone protrudes through the skin and complicates the actual fracture with an open wound. After setting the fracture, treat the wound as any other open wound unless there is arterial bleeding. Stopping the bleeding is then the priority. A closed fracture has no open wounds and the skin is intact. Follow the guidelines for immobilization, and set and splint the fracture.

*Symptoms*:

Swelling or bruising over a bone.

Deformity of an arm or leg.

Pain in the area that gets worse when the area is moved or pressure is applied.

Loss of function in the injured area.

In compound fractures, bone protruding from the skin.

There could be grating (sound and/or feeling when two ends rub together). This is called crepitus.

*Treatment:*

As with any other injury, optimally you would stabilize the victim until proper treatment or evacuation by trained professionals.

Move the broken limb as little as possible. A danger is that the broken ends of the bone could cut a blood vessel causing internal bleeding leading to shock and ultimately death. Moving the broken ends could also cause nerve damage. If the area below the break becomes numb, swollen, cool to the touch, or turns pale, and the victim shows signs of shock, a major vessel may have been severed. Rest the victim for shock, and replace lost fluids.

Only try to reset the break if help is not on the way and you are isolated.

To set the break, you are trying to relieve pain and return the limb to its anatomically correct position. This is

47

called traction. You hold upper part of the limb above the break in place, and put tension on the lower part, lining them up. If alone, you can wedge a foot or hand, and then use the other limb to push against whatever you are wedged in.

This is difficult to do in a break in the thigh as those are very strong muscles.

Once you set the break, you have to maintain the position with a splint. You should have one in your Grab-n-Go bag. If not, use anything long and solid, such as branches.

Put these on either side of the break. If it is an open fracture, keep them away from the open wound. Then securely tie in place.

For a broken leg:

Very strong muscles hold a broken thighbone (femur) in place making it difficult to maintain traction during healing. You can make an improvised traction splint using natural material as follows:

Get two forked branches or saplings at least 5 centimeters in diameter. Measure one from the patient's armpit to 7 to 10 inches past the unbroken leg. Measure the other from the groin to 7 to 10 inches past the unbroken leg. Ensure that both extend an equal distance beyond the end of the leg.

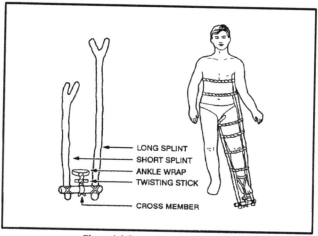

LONG SPLINT
SHORT SPLINT
ANKLE WRAP
TWISTING STICK
CROSS MEMBER

**Figure 4-6. Improvised traction splint.**

Pad the two splints. Notch the ends without forks and lash a 7 to 10 inch cross member made from a 5-centimeter diameter branch between them.

Using available material (vines, cloth, rawhide), tie the splint around the upper portion of the body and down the length of the broken leg. Follow the splinting guidelines.

With available material, fashion a wrap that will extend around the ankle, with the two free ends tied to the cross member.

Place a 4 inch by 1 inch stick in the middle of the free ends of the ankle wrap between the cross member and the foot. Using the stick, twist the material to make the traction easier.

Continue twisting until the broken leg is as long or slightly longer than the unbroken leg.

Lash the stick to maintain traction.

Over time you may lose traction because the material weakens. Check the traction periodically. If you must change or repair the splint, maintain the traction manually for a short time.

If the fracture is an open wound, but not arterial, make sure you apply pressure and stop the bleeding.

## Dislocations

A dislocation occurs in a bone joint when the bones go out of proper alignment. This tends to be very painful. It can also cause an impairment of nerve or circulatory function below the area affected.

*Symptoms*:

Visible deformity in the joint.

Swollen or discolored.

Intensely painful.

Immovable.

Limited range of motion.

*Treatment:*

Sometimes it is difficult to tell if it is a dislocation or a broken bone, so be aware of the dangers. Only try to set if there is no other choice.

Set the bones back into proper alignment. You can use several methods, but manual traction or the use of weights to pull the bones are the safest and easiest. Once performed, reduction decreases the victim's pain and allows for normal function and circulation. Without an X ray, you can judge proper alignment by the look and feel of the joint and by comparing it to the joint on the opposite side.

Immobilization is splinting the dislocation after reduction. You can use any field-expedient material for a splint or you can splint an extremity to the body.

The basic guidelines for splinting are:

Splint above and below the fracture site.

Pad splints to reduce discomfort.

Check circulation below the fracture after making each tie on the splint.

To rehabilitate the dislocation, remove the splints after 7 to 14 days. Gradually use the injured joint until fully healed.

**Sprains**

A sprain is the overstretching of a tendon or ligament. They vary in severity.

*Symptoms:*

One of the most common joints to sprain is the ankle. This is also the most dangerous in an emergency situation as it reduces mobility. To deduce if you have a sprained ankle or a broken one:

Was there a sound/feeling when it happened? If there was an audible crack, you've got a broken bone. If there was a pop, it's likely a sprain.

Is the ankle deformed or crooked? Most likely broken.

Is the ankle numb? Most likely broken.

If you cannot move the ankle at all and/or cannot put any weight on it? Broken.

*Treatment:*

When treating sprains, think RICE:

R - Rest injured area.

I - Ice for 24 hours, then heat after that.

C - Compression-wrapping and/or splinting to help stabilize. If possible, leave the boot on a sprained ankle unless circulation is compromised.

E - Elevation of the affected area.

# WATER FIRST AID

Since we can last only three days without water, it's important to understand some basics about our body and water. Water procurement is in the next section of this manual.

Over three-quarters of your body is composed of fluid. Perspiration is not the only way you lose water. We actually lose more water just by breathing. And you can't stop *that* loss. We lose around 2 to 4 cups of water a day by exhaling (16 cups equal one gallon). We lose about 2 cups via perspiration. We lose ½ to a cup just from the soles of our feet. We lose six cups via urination. When you add that up (and it wasn't easy converting all that) you lose a more than half a gallon of water a day just existing; more depending on the weather and your activity level.

Water is critical for functioning.

Dehydration results from inadequate replacement of lost body fluids. It decreases your efficiency and, if injured, increases your susceptibility to shock. Consider the following results of body fluid loss:

A 5 percent loss of body fluids results in thirst, irritability, nausea, and weakness.

A 10 percent loss results in dizziness, headache, inability to walk, and a tingling sensation in the limbs.

A 15 percent loss results in dim vision, painful urination, swollen tongue, deafness, and a numb feeling in the skin.

A loss greater than 15 percent of body fluids may result in death.

*Symptoms of dehydration are:*

Dark urine with a very strong odor. This is the one leaders must be on the lookout for.

Low urine output.

Dark, sunken eyes.

Fatigue

Emotional instability.

Loss of skin elasticity. Pinch the skin on the back of your hand and pull it up. It should immediately go back into place. If it maintains the pinched shape for a couple of seconds, then slowly settles back, you may be dehydrated.

Delayed capillary refill in fingernail beds.

Trench line down center of tongue.

Thirst. Last on the list because you are already 2 percent dehydrated by the time you crave fluids.

*Treatment*:

Replace the water as you lose it. Trying to make up a deficit is difficult in an emergency situation, and thirst is not a sign of how much water you need.

Most people cannot comfortably drink more than 1 liter of water at a time. Nor do you want to. So, even when not thirsty, drink small amounts of water at regular intervals each hour to prevent dehydration.

Drink sufficient water but don't overdo it. *Over-hydration* is a potentially fatal condition. You drink too much water for your kidneys to process. It's not just the amount, but how quickly you drink the water. Drinking too much water increases the amount of water in your blood. This dilutes the electrolytes, especially sodium. Sodium is critical in balancing the fluid inside and outside of cells. When there is an imbalance from over-hydration, sodium moves inside the cells, causing them to swell. This is particularly dangerous to your brain cells.

Thus one of the first symptoms is a headache. Nausea and vomiting are also symptoms. If it gets worse, more symptoms follow, including high blood pressure, confusion, double vision, drowsiness, difficulty breathing, muscle weakness and cramping. If not caught in time, seizures will occur, brain damage, coma and even death.

A dangerous thing about hyponatremia (what this is called) is that it can be confused with dehydration and people can force the victim to drink more water. Extreme sports athletes are at risk for this, as well people during a heat wave. Without access to special medications, primary treatment for this to stop the water intake. If symptoms are not extreme, try to balance out the sodium with a sports that contains sodium.

If you are under physical and mental stress or subject to severe conditions, increase your water intake. Drink enough liquids to maintain a urine output of at least half a quart every 24 hours.

In any situation where food intake is low, drink 6 to 8 quarters of water per day. In an extreme climate, especially an arid one, the average person can lose 2.5 to 3.5 quarts of water *per hour*. In this type of climate, you should drink 14 to 30 quarts of water per day.

With the loss of water there is also a loss of electrolytes (body salts). The average diet can usually keep up with these losses but in an extreme situation or illness, additional sources need to be provided. A mixture of 0.25 teaspoon of salt to 1 liter of water will provide a concentration that the body tissues can readily absorb.

Make sure you drink water while eating. This aids in digestion. In adverse conditions, particularly cold and wet environments, a leader must force his or her people to drink water, even when they don't feel like it.

Of all the First Aid problems encountered in a survival situation, the loss of water is the most preventable. Acquiring water is a different problem we will deal with shortly.

*Dehydration Treatment*:

For dehydration that is short of heat stroke:

Drink two quarts of water, juice or sports drinks in 2 to 4 hours, not all at once. Small sips every few minutes work best.

If vomiting, try ice chips, popsicles and small sips.

If also suffering from diarrhea, stay away from using sports drinks as the sugar can make it worse.

**Heat Stroke**

The breakdown of the body's heat regulatory system causes a heat stroke. It occurs when your core body temperature goes to 104 degrees. Other heat injuries, such as cramps or dehydration, do not always precede a heatstroke.

Heat stroke is extremely dangerous. As with all other dangerous conditions, call 911, evacuate or get profession help if possible.

Heat stroke can kill or cause serious damage to the brain and other organs. It happens after prolonged exposure to high temperatures in combination with dehydration.

*Symptoms*:

Swollen, beet-red face.

Reddened whites of eyes.

Victim not sweating. Red, hot and dry skin.

Unconsciousness or delirium, which can cause pallor, a bluish color to lips and nail beds (cyanosis), and cool skin.

*Treatment:*

Fan air over the victim while wetting skin with water.

Apply ice packs to the armpits, groin, neck, and back. These areas have more blood vessels on average, so cooling them can reduce the body temperature.

Immerse the patient in a shower or tub of cool water. Or a stream or lake.

Be sure to wet the victim's head. Heat loss through the scalp is great.

Expect, during cooling:

Vomiting.

Diarrhea.

Struggling.

Shivering.

Shouting.

Prolonged unconsciousness.

Rebound heatstroke within 48 hours.

Cardiac arrest; be ready to perform CPR.

Note: Treat for dehydration with lightly salted water.

# COLD WEATHER INJURIES

### Hypothermia

This occurs when the body's core temperature falls to 95 degrees F or cooler. It is the opposite of heat stroke. Wind chill multiplies the effect of cold. Wind chill is the effect of moving air on exposed flesh. Wind always exacerbates the situation, which is why your outer garment should not only be water resistant, but wind resistant. A key in building shelter is to get out of the wind.

Here is a handy chart showing the effect of wind chill.

## Wind Chill Chart

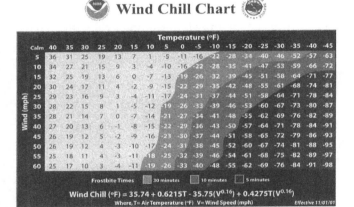

| Wind (mph) | Temperature (°F) | | | | | | | | | | | | | | | | | |
|---|---|---|---|---|---|---|---|---|---|---|---|---|---|---|---|---|---|---|
| Calm | 40 | 35 | 30 | 25 | 20 | 15 | 10 | 5 | 0 | -5 | -10 | -15 | -20 | -25 | -30 | -35 | -40 | -45 |
| 5 | 36 | 31 | 25 | 19 | 13 | 7 | 1 | -5 | -11 | -16 | -22 | -28 | -34 | -40 | -46 | -52 | -57 | -63 |
| 10 | 34 | 27 | 21 | 15 | 9 | 3 | -4 | -10 | -16 | -22 | -28 | -35 | -41 | -47 | -53 | -59 | -66 | -72 |
| 15 | 32 | 25 | 19 | 13 | 6 | 0 | -7 | -13 | -19 | -26 | -32 | -39 | -45 | -51 | -58 | -64 | -71 | -77 |
| 20 | 30 | 24 | 17 | 11 | 4 | -2 | -9 | -15 | -22 | -29 | -35 | -42 | -48 | -55 | -61 | -68 | -74 | -81 |
| 25 | 29 | 23 | 16 | 9 | 3 | -4 | -11 | -17 | -24 | -31 | -37 | -44 | -51 | -58 | -64 | -71 | -78 | -84 |
| 30 | 28 | 22 | 15 | 8 | 1 | -5 | -12 | -19 | -26 | -33 | -39 | -46 | -53 | -60 | -67 | -73 | -80 | -87 |
| 35 | 28 | 21 | 14 | 7 | 0 | -7 | -14 | -21 | -27 | -34 | -41 | -48 | -55 | -62 | -69 | -76 | -82 | -89 |
| 40 | 27 | 20 | 13 | 6 | -1 | -8 | -15 | -22 | -29 | -36 | -43 | -50 | -57 | -64 | -71 | -78 | -84 | -91 |
| 45 | 26 | 19 | 12 | 5 | -2 | -9 | -16 | -23 | -30 | -37 | -44 | -51 | -58 | -65 | -72 | -79 | -86 | -93 |
| 50 | 26 | 19 | 12 | 4 | -3 | -10 | -17 | -24 | -31 | -38 | -45 | -52 | -60 | -67 | -74 | -81 | -88 | -95 |
| 55 | 25 | 18 | 11 | 4 | -3 | -11 | -18 | -25 | -32 | -39 | -46 | -54 | -61 | -68 | -75 | -82 | -89 | -97 |
| 60 | 25 | 17 | 10 | 3 | -4 | -11 | -19 | -26 | -33 | -40 | -48 | -55 | -62 | -69 | -76 | -84 | -91 | -98 |

Frostbite Times   30 minutes   10 minutes   5 minutes

$$\text{Wind Chill (°F)} = 35.74 + 0.6215T - 35.75(V^{0.16}) + 0.4275T(V^{0.16})$$

Where, T= Air Temperature (°F)  V= Wind Speed (mph)          Effective 11/01/01

Getting wet accelerates the onset of progression of hypothermia since the body loses heat 25 times faster in cold water than in cold air. Since it affects the core temperature this means that the brain, heart, lungs and other vital organs are affected.

Some people are more susceptible to hypothermia: the elderly, children, and those under the influence of alcohol. Children and thin people lose body heat more quickly.

Cold Water Survival Times

| Water Temperature | Becomes Unconscious | Time to Death |
|---|---|---|
| 32.5 F | Under 15 minutes | Under 45 minutes |
| 32.5 to 40 F | 15 to 30 minutes | 30 to 90 minutes |
| 40 to 50 F | 30 to 60 minutes | 1 to 3 hours |
| 50 to 60 F | 1 to 2 hours | 1 to 6 hours |
| 60 to 70 F | 2 to 7 hours | 2 to 40 hours |
| 70 to 80 F | 3 to 12 hours | 3 hours to indefinite |

As you can see, even relatively mild water temperatures of 70 to 80 F can cause hypothermia. While those times are for immersion, getting wet and not being to get to a shelter outdoors also causes hypothermia. As does simply staying cold even if you're not wet.

*Prevention:*

Stay hydrated.

Stay fueled; eat properly and sufficient calories for the energy expended. In Winter Warfare training, we upped our rations, knowing what we would be facing.

Seek shelter. Get out of the elements if possible. This is a situation where shelter can become more important than water or food, as being hypothermic outdoors for 3 hours can kill.

In your Grab-n-Go bag you have a wool hat and gloves. You lose 40 to 45 percent of body heat from an unprotected head and even more from the unprotected neck, wrist, and ankles. These areas of the body are good radiators of heat and have very little insulating fat.

Avoid sweating in a cold weather environment. That's causing yourself to become wet.

*Symptoms:*

Shivering. Confusion. Uncoordinated actions.

*Treatment:*

Get into shelter.

Build a fire if you don't have a shelter.

Remove wet clothing and replace with dry or put in a sleeping bag or cover with blankets.

Sip on a warm beverage (nothing with caffeine or alcohol).

Do gentle exercises.

Get in your sleeping bag. If necessary, have someone who is not hypothermic share it, to give their body heat.

If you have hand warmers, put them in the same place ice would go for heat stroke: necks, armpits and groin.

### Frostbite

Frostbite is the freezing of your external blood vessels and the flesh surrounding them. The most common places for this to occur are exposed skin in the ears, nose and cheeks. Also, toes, feet, fingers and hands.

*Prevention*: Proper clothing, worn correctly in layers, as described in *Prepare Now-Survive Later*.

Wearing gloves all the time.

Use a buddy system to check each other for symptoms.

Maintain circulation by twitching and wrinkling the skin on your face making faces. Warm with your hands. If outdoors in cold weather for an extended period of time, men shouldn't shave. Doing so removes natural oils that protect the skin.

Wiggle and move your ears. Warm with your hands.

Move your hands inside your gloves. Warm by placing your hands close to your body.

Move your feet and wiggle your toes inside your boots. Changing your socks often to keep them dry and clean.

*Symptoms*:

Stinging pain that turns into numbness. You might not even feel the pain, depending on the circumstances and what else is going on in an emergency.

The skin becomes cold to the touch and white spots develop.

*Treatment*:

As with everything else, medical attention ASAP if possible; frostbite can cause permanent injuries and even amputation.

If medical attention isn't available within the next two to three hours, get into shelter or build a fire. Submerge body parts in water that is between 104 and 108; tepid water, not hot. Submerging in hot water will cause extreme pain and even shock. Do not expose frostbite to flame. This tepid water will cool quickly, drawing the cold from the body. Change it often.

When drying frostbite injuries pat them. Don't rub. Rubbing causes more damage.

Blisters may appear. Do not pop or lance them as that increases the chances of infection. Apply a loose sterile dressing over the affected area.

# FOOD

Although you can live several weeks without food, you need an adequate amount to stay healthy. Without food your mental and physical capabilities will deteriorate rapidly, and you will become weak. Food replenishes the substances that your body uses and provides energy. Food provides vitamins, minerals, salts, and other elements essential to good health.

The two basic sources of food are plants and animals (including fish). In varying degrees both provide the calories, carbohydrates, fats, and proteins needed for normal daily body functions.

Calories are a measure of heat and potential energy. The average person needs roughly 2,000 calories per day to function at a minimum level. In extreme situations we can do to 800 calories but not for long. I recommend 2,400 calories as your planning baseline in *Prepare Now-Survive Later*.

*Plant Foods:*

These foods provide carbohydrates—the main source of energy. Many plants provide enough protein to keep the body at normal efficiency. Although plants may not provide a balanced diet, they will sustain you even in the arctic, where meat's heat-producing qualities are normally essential. Many plant foods such as nuts and seeds will give you enough protein and oils for normal efficiency. Roots, green vegetables, and plant food containing natural sugar will provide calories and carbohydrates that give the body natural energy.

The food value of plants becomes more and more important if you are eluding the enemy or if you are in an area where wildlife is scarce.

You can dry plants by wind, air, sun, or fire. This retards spoilage so that you can store or carry the plant food with you to use when needed.

You can obtain plants more easily and more quietly than meat.

*Animal Foods:*

Meat is more nourishing than plant food. In fact, it may even be more readily available in some places. However, to get meat, you need to know the habits of, and how to capture, the various wildlife.

To satisfy your immediate food needs, first seek the more abundant and more easily obtained wildlife, such as insects, crustaceans, mollusks, fish, and reptiles. These can satisfy your immediate hunger while you are preparing traps and snares for larger game.

Food procurement will be covered shortly.

# BITES AND STINGS

Insects and related pests are hazards in everyday life, not just emergency situations. They often carry disease. In some cases, bites and stings can be fatal because of poison or a severe allergic reactions in some individuals.

*Ticks* can carry and transmit diseases, such as Rocky Mountain spotted fever common in many parts of the United States. Ticks also transmit the Lyme disease.

*Mosquitoes* may carry malaria, dengue, and many other diseases.

*Flies* can spread disease from contact with infectious sources. They are causes of sleeping sickness, typhoid, cholera, and dysentery.

*Fleas* can transmit plague.

*Lice* can transmit typhus and relapsing fever.

The best way to avoid the complications of insect bites and stings is to keep immunizations (including booster shots) up-to-date, avoid insect-infested areas, use netting and insect repellent, and wear all clothing properly.

If you get bitten or stung, do not scratch the bite or sting, it might become infected. Inspect your body at least once a day to ensure there are no insects attached to you. If you find ticks attached to your body, cover them with a substance, such as Vaseline, heavy oil, or tree sap, that will cut off their air supply. Without air, the tick releases its hold, and you can remove it. Take care to remove the whole tick. Use tweezers if you have them. Grasp the tick where the mouth parts are attached to the skin. Do not squeeze the tick's body. Wash your hands after touching the tick. Clean the tick wound daily until healed.

### Bee and Wasp Stings

If stung by a bee, immediately remove the stinger and venom sac, if attached, by scraping with a fingernail or a knife blade. Do not squeeze or grasp the stinger or venom sac, as squeezing will force more venom into the wound.

Wash the sting site thoroughly with soap and water to lessen the chance of a secondary infection.

If you are allergic, you should always have your epipen auto-injector with you.

**Spider Bites and Scorpion Stings**

The black widow spider is identified by a red hourglass on its abdomen. Only the female bites and it has a neurotoxic venom. The initial pain is not severe, but severe local pain rapidly develops. The pain gradually spreads over the entire body and settles in the abdomen and legs. Abdominal cramps and progressive nausea, vomiting, and a rash may occur. Weakness, tremors, sweating, and salivation may occur. Anaphylactic reactions can occur. Symptoms begin to regress after several hours and are usually gone in a few days.

Threat for shock. Be ready to perform CPR. Clean and dress the bite area to reduce the risk of infection. An antivenom is available.

The brown house spider or brown recluse spider is a small, light brown spider identified by a dark brown violin on its back. You usually are no aware you've been bitten at the time because there is little pain. Within a few hours a painful red area with a mottled cyanotic center appears. Necrosis does not occur in all bites, but usually in 3 to 4 days, a star-shaped, firm area of deep purple discoloration appears at the bite site. The area turns dark and mummified in a week or two. The margins separate and the scab falls off, leaving an open ulcer. Secondary infection and regional swollen lymph glands usually become visible at this stage. The outstanding characteristic of the brown recluse bite is an ulcer that does not heal but persists for weeks or months. In addition to the ulcer, there is often a systemic reaction that is serious and may lead to death. Speaking from experience, a brown recluse bite goes un-noticed, but eventually is painful and noticeable.

Reactions (fever, chills, joint pain, vomiting, and a generalized rash) occur chiefly in children or debilitated persons.

Tarantulas are large, hairy spiders found mainly in the tropics. Most do not inject venom, but some South American species do. They have large fangs. If bitten, pain and bleeding are certain, and infection is likely. Treat a tarantula bite as for any open wound, and try to prevent infection. If symptoms of poisoning appear, treat as for the bite of the black widow spider.

Scorpions are all poisonous to a greater or lesser degree. There are two different reactions, depending on the species: Severe local reaction only, with pain and swelling around the area of the sting. Possible prickly sensation around the mouth and a thick-feeling tongue.

Severe systemic reaction, with little or no visible local reaction. Local pain may be present. Systemic reaction includes respiratory difficulties, thick-feeling tongue, body spasms, drooling, gastric distention, double vision, blindness, involuntary rapid movement of the eyeballs, involuntary urination and defecation, and heart failure. Death is rare, occurring mainly in children and adults with high blood pressure or illnesses.

Treat scorpion stings as you would a black widow bite.

**Snakebites**

The chance of a snakebite in an emergency situation is rather small, if you are familiar with the various types of snakes and their habitats. However, it could happen and you should know how to treat a snakebite. Deaths from snakebites are rare. More than one-half of snakebite victims have little or no poisoning, and only about one-quarter develop serious systemic poisoning.

The primary concern in the treatment of snakebite is to limit the amount of eventual tissue destruction around the bite area.

A bite wound, regardless of the type of animal that inflicted it, can become infected from bacteria in the animal's mouth. With nonpoisonous as well as poisonous snakebites, this local infection is responsible for a large part of the residual damage that results.

Snake venoms not only contain poisons that attack the victim's central nervous system (neurotoxins) and blood circulation (hemotoxins), but also digestive enzymes (cytotoxins) to aid in digesting their prey. These poisons can cause a very large area of tissue death, leaving a large open wound. This condition could lead to the need for eventual amputation if not treated.

Shock and panic in a person bitten by a snake can also affect the person's recovery. Excitement, hysteria, and panic can speed up the circulation, causing the body to absorb the toxin quickly. Signs of shock could occur within the first 30 minutes after the bite.

Before you start treating a snakebite, determine whether the snake was poisonous or nonpoisonous. There are four types of poisonous snakes in North America. In your Area Study you should have determined if any are endemic to your area.

Overall, venomous snakes have a triangular head (not so much on the Coral), while non-venomous have more spoon-shaped heads.

Cottonmouths: elliptical pupils and range in color from black to green. They have a white stripe along the sides of their head. They are normally found in or around water. The young have a bright yellow tail. They usually are alone.

Rattlesnakes: A triangular head with elliptical eyes. And of course, a rattle on their tail.

Copperheads: Brightly colored from coppery brown to bright orange, silver-pink and peach. The young also have yellow tails.

Coral snakes: Several non-venomous snakes look like Coral snakes. They have a distinctive coloring, with black, yellow, and red bands. They have a yellow head with a black band over their nose. They are extremely shy and rarely bite. The difference between a Coral and a King Snake is: "red on black, venom lack. Red on yellow, deadly fellow."

Bites from a nonpoisonous snake will show rows of teeth. Bites from a poisonous snake may have rows of teeth showing, but will have one or more distinctive puncture marks caused by fang penetration.

Symptoms of a poisonous bite may be spontaneous bleeding from the nose and anus, blood in the urine, pain at the site of the bite, and swelling at the site of the bite within a few minutes or up to 2 hours later.

Breathing difficulty, paralysis, weakness, twitching, and numbness are also signs of neurotoxic venoms. These signs usually appear 1.5 to 2 hours after the bite.

If you determine that a poisonous snake bit an individual, take the following steps:

Reassure the victim and keep him still.

Remove watches, rings, bracelets, or other constricting items.

Clean the bite area.

Maintain an airway (especially if bitten near the face or neck) and be prepared to administer mouth-to-mouth resuscitation or CPR.

Use a constricting band between the wound and the heart. Immobilize the site.

Remove the poison as soon as possible by using a mechanical suction device or by squeezing.

**Do not**

Give the victim alcoholic beverages or tobacco products.

Give morphine or other central nervous system (CNS) depressors.

Make any deep cuts at the bite site. Cutting opens capillaries that in turn open a direct route into the blood stream for venom and infection.

Put your hands on your face or rub your eyes, as venom may be on your hands. Venom may cause blindness.

Break open the large blisters that form around the bite site.

After caring for the victim as described above, take the following actions to minimize local effects:

If infection appears, keep the wound open and clean.

Use heat after 24 to 48 hours to help prevent the spread of local infection. Heat also helps to draw out an infection.

Keep the wound covered with a dry, sterile dressing.

Have the victim drink large amounts of fluids until the infection is gone.

Snakes usually avoid people. Rattlers never really concerned me; we used to eat them and they do taste like chicken. Where snakes can be dangerous is in the water. Hitting a nest of water moccasins can be deadly.

# PERSONAL HYGEINE

During a high moderate or extreme emergency, you might go weeks, months and longer in uncomfortable circumstances, whether in the wild or in crowded centers. Hygiene isn't just a matter of politeness or comfort, but it helps prevent infection and disease and becomes critical in such circumstances.

Wash yourself when possible, paying particular attention to the feet, armpits, crotch, hands, and hair. Those are primary areas for infection and infestation.

If water is scarce, and the weather permitting, strip down and expose your body to the air for a little while, without getting sunburned.

*Keep Your Hands Clean.* This goes even in non-emergency situations. Germs on your hands can infect food and wounds. Wash your hands after handling any material that is likely to carry germs, after visiting the latrine, after caring for the sick, and before handling any food, food utensils, or drinking water. Keep your fingernails closely trimmed and clean.

*Keep Your Hair Clean.* Your hair can become a haven for bacteria or fleas, lice, and other parasites. Keeping your hair clean, combed, and trimmed helps you avoid this danger.

*Keep Your Clothing Clean.* Keep your clothing and bedding as clean as possible to reduce the chance of skin infection as well as to decrease the danger of parasitic infestation. Clean your outer clothing whenever it becomes soiled. Wear clean underclothing and socks as much as possible. If water is scarce, clean your clothing by shaking, airing, and sunning it for 2 hours. If you are using a sleeping bag, turn it inside out after each use, fluff it, and air it.

*Keep Your Teeth Clean.* Thoroughly clean your mouth and teeth with a toothbrush at least once each day. If you don't have a toothbrush, make a chewing stick. Find a twig. Chew one end of the stick to separate the fibers. Now brush your teeth thoroughly. Another way is to wrap a clean strip of cloth around your fingers and rub your teeth with it to wipe away food particles. You can also brush your teeth with small amounts of sand, baking soda, salt, or soap. Then rinse your mouth. Flossing your teeth with string or fiber helps oral hygiene.

*Take Care of Your Feet.* To prevent serious foot problems, break in your shoes before wearing them. Wash and massage your feet daily. Trim your toe-nails straight across. Wear an insole and the proper size of dry socks. Powder and check your feet daily for blisters. If you get a small blister, do not open it. An intact blister is safe from infection. Apply a padding material around the blister to relieve pressure and reduce friction. If the blister bursts, treat it as an open wound. Clean and dress it daily and pad around it. Leave large blisters intact.

*Keep Camp Site Clean.* Do not soil the ground in the camp site area with urine or feces. Use latrines, if available. When latrines are not available, dig "cat holes" and cover the waste. Collect drinking water upstream from the camp site. Purify all water.

# WATER PROCUREMENT

A stockpile of water was your first priority in *Prepare Now-Survive Later*. Your baseline requirement is a gallon a day, per person. This is variable depending on environment and what you are doing.

### Water
On average, we can survive three days without water versus three weeks without food.

Over three-quarters of your body is composed of fluid. Perspiration is not the only way you lose water. We actually lose more water just by breathing. And you can't stop *that* loss. We lose around 2 to 4 cups of water a day by exhaling (16 cups equal one gallon). We lose about 2 cups via perspiration. We lose ½ to a cup just from the soles of our feet. We lose six cups via urination. When you add that up (and it wasn't easy converting all that) you lose a more than half a gallon of water a day just existing; more depending on the weather and your activity level.

Water is critical for functioning. A 5% drop in body fluid will cause a 25% drop in energy level. A 15% drop will cause death. Even in normal day-to-day living, it is estimated that 80% of people are fatigued simply because they are chronically dehydrated.

What water resources did you list in your Area Study? Which of those are accessible now?

# WARNING!
## Most Water in Nature is Unsafe to Drink

The spread of Giardia has made most water sources that you used to be able to trust, unsafe. Whatever purification system you use, make sure it will get rid of Giardia. Giardia is spread through animal dropping. If you get this bug, it will seriously degrade you physically and reduce your ability to survive.

By drinking non-potable water you may contract diseases or swallow organisms that can harm you. Examples of such diseases or organisms are—

*Dysentery.* Severe, prolonged diarrhea with bloody stools, fever, and weakness.

*Cholera and typhoid.* You may be susceptible to these diseases regardless of inoculations.

*Flukes.* Stagnant, polluted water—especially in tropical areas—often contains blood flukes. If you swallow flukes, they will bore into the bloodstream, live as parasites, and cause disease.

*Leeches.* If you swallow a leech, it can hook onto the throat passage or inside the nose. It will suck blood, create a wound, and move to another area. Each bleeding wound may become infected.


We have te problem of industrial and chemical pollution. You have little idea what run off is going into the water. So stay away from water:

That is near roads. As a corollary to this, ever notice the sheen on a road as rain starts? That's all the oil and other pollutants in the road lifting up. This is the most dangerous time for traction.

Don't drink downstream or river of factories that discharge into the water, sewage systems that discharge, mines or, frankly sites of major human habitation.

Don't drink water draining out of utilized farmland. You don't want to know what they're spraying in that soil and on those crops.

If you are in an area that has been flooded (aka Katrina), consider all water sources affected by the flooding to be contaminated, even if they were previously considered drinkable.

You have to assume that any water that isn't marked as potable (drinkable) is contaminated. Even in the deepest forest, there is a chance the water is tainted. Always stay on the safe side, because contracting Giardia is no fun at all and cholera can be fatal.

## Water sources in your home

The hot water heater contains a considerable amount. There is a drain at the bottom. Make sure you have something to collect the water in, open the drain, then open a faucet to complete the water circuit. (Make sure, if not already off, that you turn off the gas/power to the heater before working on it, throw the circuit breaker. If the power/gas is already off and comes on, make sure you immediately refill the heater before you turn it back on or else it can overheat.)

The water pipes in your house can be drained of the water in them.

The toilet tank (not the toilet bowl) contains fresh water. Get over it and use it.

A swimming pool or hot tub contains non-potable water you can use for washing, not drinking unless you make it potable.

If you have adequate warning, you should fill every available container with potable water. Also fill all tubs and sinks.

*There are items in your house that can be used to purify water*:

Chlorine Bleach. Standard bleach is 5% chlorine. If the strength is not known go with ten drops per quart or liter for clear water, double that for murky water)

### DISINFECTING WATER

| Available Chlorine Concentrate | Drops per Quart/Gallon of Clear Water (a drop is $1/8^{th}$ teaspoon) | Drops per Liter of Clear Water |
|---|---|---|
| 1.00% to 2.00% Chlorine Concentrate | 10 per quart, 40 per gallon | 10 per liter |
| Regular to Ultra Strength 5.25% to 6.00% | 2 per quart, 8 per gallon | 2 per liter |
| | Drops per Quart/Gallon of Cloudy Water | Drops per Quart/Gallon of Cloudy Water |
| 1.00% to 2.00% Chlorine Concentrate | 20 per quart, 80 per gallon | 20 per liter |
| Regular to Ultra Strength 5.25% to 6.00% | 4 per quart, 16 per gallon | 4 per liter |
| Stir the mixture well | Let it stand for 30 minutes | |

### BOILING WATER

| | |
|---|---|
| Filter to remove impurities | Use coffee filter, towel, etc. |
| Bring to boil | Continue for one minute |
| Bring to boil for one minute and | Add 1 minute at boil for every 1,000 feet of altitude |

# Water sources in nature

Warning! Purify any water that you are not positive is drinkable.

*Rainwater* collected in clean containers is usually safe for drinking. This is the quickest and most effective way to gather potable water.

*Lakes, ponds, swamps, springs, streams*. Must be purified regardless of how clear and clean it looks. This is especially true if it is anywhere near human settlements.

*Underground water*: Muddy ground indicates a water supply. You can filter the muddy water or dig down about a foot and gather what collects. It still must be purified.

*Snow and ice:* Are as pure as the water from which they came, this is particularly true for ice. Do not eat snow or ice without melting first, as doing so will reduce your core body temperature and actually lead to dehydration more than hydration.

*Green bamboo thickets* are a source of fresh water. Water from green bamboo is clear and odorless. To get the water, bend a green bamboo stalk, tie it down, and cut off the top. The water will drip freely during the night and collect. Old, cracked bamboo may contain water. Bamboo is a lot more common than you realize. When you did your Area Study, this is something you should have looked for: all the sources of water that you might not have considered before.

*Morning dew* can provide water. Use an absorbent cloth (this is one case where cotton isn't rotten) or a handful of long grass and wick up moisture that has condense. You can also tie rags or tufts of fine grass around your ankles and walk through dew-covered grass before sunrise. As the cloth, rags or grass tufts absorb the dew, wring the water into a container. Repeat the process until you have a supply of water or until the dew is gone. This water is consider potable (unless you collect it off of poison ivy or recently fertilized/sprayed grass, etc.)

*Banana/plantain trees*: Cut down the tree, leaving a stump about a foot high. Scoop out the center, leaving a bowl shaped hollow. Water from the roots will come and being the fill the hollow. The first several fillings will be bitter, but then it was become more palatable. This can supply water for up to four days. If you are going to re-use, cover it to keep insects and bugs out.

*Tropical vines*: Cut a notch as high as you can reach. Do not drink if it is sticky, milky or bitter-tasting.

*Coconuts*: The milk from unripe (green) coconuts. The milk from mature coconuts contains a laxative.

### WARNING! Do not drink the following:

| | |
|---|---|
| Seawater | It is 4 percent salt. It takes 2 quarts of body fluids to rid the body of the waste produced by 1 quart of seawater. You are actually dehydrating yourself twice as fast |
| Blood | Is considered a food since it's salty, therefore requiring additional body fluid to process. Also may transmit disease. |
| Urine | 2% salt and contains harmful body wastes. |
| Alcoholic beverages | Dehydrate you and cloud your judgement. |
| Sea ice | Same as seawater. |

# Ways to Purify Water

*Grab-n-Go bag*: You have: Survival straw. Survival filter. Water purification tablets. Use those sparingly if you can find potable water or can purify by other means. You also have at least one water container. Check the instructions on the filters and tablets and use properly.

If the water you find is muddy, stagnant, and/or foul smelling, you can clear the water by placing it in a container and letting it stand for 12 hours. Or by passing it through cloth multiple times. Or through sand. But these procedures only clear the water and make it more palatable. You will still have to purify it.

*Boiling*: Minimum one minute at boil at sea level. Add one minute for each thousand feet you are above sea level in altitude. You can get your altitude off your contour map.

*Solar water disinfection (SoDis)*: Given the proliferation of water bottles and the fact you probably have some in your Grab-n-Go bag, car, home, etc. this is a particularly effective method.

Find a clean, clear plastic bottle no more than three liters (1 liter is slightly more than one quart). It needs to be a PET bottle. You can tell by looking on the bottom. Most will say if they are PET or PETE. Otherwise it will have a number. You want a #1. Any other number is a different kind of plastic. The narrower the bottle, the better for solar penetration.

Fill it three quarters full with clear water, or water you have filtered through sand or whatever you have available.

Shake the bottle in order to get as much oxygen as possible into the water.

Fill the rest of the bottle and replace the lid.

Place the bottle in direct sunlight for six to eight hours. You can increase the efficiency by placing the bottle on a reflective surface such as metal or aluminum foil.

If you have to move, hang the bottle on the outside of your pack.

If it isn't sunny out (yeah, you in the Pacific Northwest) or the water is cloudy, leave it in the light for at least two full days. Really, if you live in a cloudy area like the Pacific Northwest get a water filter. In fact, no matter where you live, get a water filter. SODIS is only for extreme situations where there is no other options. Considering you can pretty much find empty plastic bottles pretty much anywhere, including the middle of the Pacific Ocean (alas Ancient Mariner, this does not convert salt water), it's a useful one to know.

How SODIS works: The sunlight treats the water through three ways, all involved radiation.

UVA reacts with the oxygen dissolved in the water to produce a highly reactive form with free radicals and hydrogen peroxide, which kills microorganisms.

UVA interferes with the reproductive cycle of bacteria by crippling their DNA.

The sunlight heats the water and once it gets it above 122 degrees, the disinfection works three times faster.

Like anything else, the combined effect of the three is cumulative. However, this technique DOES NOT remove chemical contamination.

Also, it works better in central latitudes where sunlight is not angled so much. Optimum is 35 degrees latitude north and south.

The plastic bottle should be as new as possible, not colored, and as free of scratches as possible. Glass bottles can be used but only as a last resort as they are not as effective.

The thinner the bottle, the better, to allow the sunlight to penetrate.

Of note, SODIS is being used in various places around the world to produce potable water, due to the lack of treated water.

*Aboveground Still:* To make the aboveground still, you need a sunny slope on which to place the still, a clear plastic bag, green leafy vegetation, and a small rock (Figure 6-6).

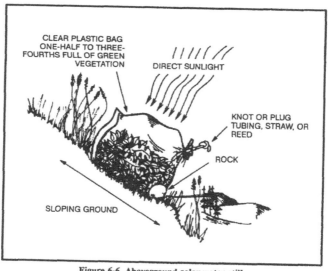

**Figure 6-6. Aboveground solar water still.**

To make the still—

Fill the bag with air by turning the opening into the breeze or by "scooping" air into the bag. Fill the plastic bag half to three-fourths full of green leafy vegetation. Be sure to remove all hard sticks or sharp spines that might puncture the bag.

Place a small rock or similar item in the bag.

Close the bag and tie the mouth securely as close to the end of the bag as possible to keep the maximum amount of airspace. If you have a piece of tubing, a small straw, or a hollow reed, insert one end in the mouth of the bag before you tie it securely. Then tie off or plug the tubing so that air will not escape. This tubing will allow you to drain out condensed water without untying the bag.

Place the bag, mouth downhill, on a slope in full sunlight. Position the mouth of the bag slightly higher than the low point in the bag.

Settle the bag in place so that the rock works itself into the low point in the bag.

To get the condensed water from the still, loosen the tie around the bag's mouth and tip the bag so that the water collected around the rock will drain out. Then retie the mouth securely and reposition the still to allow further condensation.

Change the vegetation in the bag after extracting most of the water from it. This will ensure maximum output of water.

*Belowground Still*: To make a belowground still, you need a digging tool, a container, a clear plastic sheet, a drinking tube, and a rock (Figure 6-7).

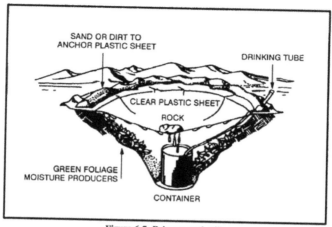

**Figure 6-7. Belowground still.**

Select a site where you believe the soil will contain moisture (such as a dry stream bed or a low spot where rainwater has collected). The soil at this site should be easy to dig, and sunlight must hit the site most of the day.

To construct the still:

Dig a bowl-shaped hole about 1 meter across and 60 centimeters deep.

Dig a sump in the center of the hole. The sump's depth and perimeter will depend on the size of the container that you have to place in it. The bottom of the sump should allow the container to stand upright. Anchor the tubing to the container's bottom by forming a loose over-hand knot in the tubing.

Place the container upright in the sump.

Extend the unanchored end of the tubing up, over, and beyond the lip of the hole.

Place the plastic sheet over the hole, covering its edges with soil to hold it in place.

Place a rock in the center of the plastic sheet.

Lower the plastic sheet into the hole until it is about 40 centimeters below ground level. It now forms an inverted cone with the rock at its apex. Make sure that the cone's apex is directly over your container. Also make sure the plastic cone does not touch the sides of the hole because the earth will absorb the condensed water.

Put more soil on the edges of the plastic to hold it securely in place and to prevent the loss of moisture.

Plug the tube when not in use so that the moisture will not evaporate.

You can drink water without disturbing the still by using the tube as a straw.

You may want to use plants in the hole as a moisture source. If so, dig out additional soil from the sides of the hole to form a slope on which to place the plants. Then proceed as above.

If polluted water is your only moisture source, dig a small trough outside the hole about 25 centimeters from the still's lip (Figure 6-8). Dig the trough about 25 centimeters deep and 8 centimeters wide. Pour the polluted water in the trough. Be sure you do not spill any polluted water around the rim of the hole where the plastic sheet touches the soil. The trough holds the polluted water and the soil filters it as the still draws it. The water then condenses on the plastic and drains into the container. This process works extremely well when your only water source is salt water. *(Do this only if you have no other option!)*

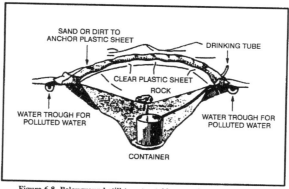

Figure 6-8. Belowground still to get potable water from polluted water.

You will need at least three stills to meet your individual daily water intake needs.

*Some rules of thumb if things are extreme and you must drink without time or ability to purify:*

Running water is better than still water.

Water coming out of a spring is better than running water.

Clear water is usually better than cloudy or discolored water (but only in an emergency as you can't see the bugs that will make you sick).

Avoid water that has algae in it.

Avoid swamp or marshland water.

In an extreme survival system when you have gone into Scavenge mode, find an abandoned house that has a water system. Find the filters for the purification system. In my current house, my kitchen sink has a three filter system that could be cannibalized and used. The key is that it requires pressure to push water through the system. But gravity provides pressure, slowly but surely.

Make sure you clearly mark and separate potable from non-potable water containers. Never, ever, mix the two.

Quite frankly, from a large Area Study of the entire world environment, potable water is becoming the most valuable resource and will soon outstrip even oil as the most precious.

I predict some future wars will be fought over access to drinkable water.

## Scavenge

Full, unopened, water bottles are everywhere in our civilization. Don't just check stores. Homes. Businesses. Vending machines. Inside cars and trucks. More under the section on Scavenge.

Look around. Listen. Smell. Watch animals. They need water.

## Sustain

A non-stop source of drinking should be your priority in finding a place to live. There are easily defendable locales such as an island or a prison, but do they have water?

### The Rule of Three

You can survive three minutes without air.

You can survive three hours without a regulated body temperature.

You can survive three days, depending on environment, without water.

You can survive three weeks without food.

# FOOD PROCUREMENT

Food is not an issue for mild emergencies. We can survive for several weeks without food. Since you have your supplies in your house and your Grab-n-Go bags ready, you are able to live off your stockpile for a while.

Your baseline in your house is 3 days non-perishable. The same for your Grab-n-Go bag. That gives you six days. Your ERP should more, if you stocked it. There is also food in your car.

On top of that, you have your everyday pantry and refrigerator.

If the power goes out, use the food from your refrigerator first, starting with the freezer.

As we move from mild into moderate emergencies, and the time gets longer, food will start to become more of an issue.

Disclaimer: If you want to learn how hunt, trap, fish, skin animals, butcher them, etc. *after* an emergency or disaster happens is probably not the best time. The smarter plan is to have someone on your survival team who knows how to do this or learn to do it beforehand. I will give some basics from which you can expand.

Food is an area where people will go into scavenge mode and, if resourceful, can stay there for a long time. Long enough, more importantly, to begin planting crops. As we will note in Sustain, if civilization collapses, we will follow the historical path our ancestors did in building back up: after scavenging no longer works, those who are still alive, will become hunter/gatherers, while some will jump right to farming. The danger with farming is that it makes you stationery, which makes you a target for scavengers.

It's a vicious formula.

The same with having domesticated animals. Great idea, and they are moveable, but they are also targets.

*Extreme emergency food considerations:*

I noted that a person can go three weeks without food. That, however, is really stretching it. I've gone eight days without food; interestingly I stopped feeling hungry after a bit. However, the ability to function begins to degrade.

When our output exceeds our caloric intake these are the symptoms:

-physical weakness

-confusion, poor judgment, and disorientation

-weakened immune system

-inability to maintain body temperature which can lead to hypothermia, heat exhaustion/stroke.

The Coast Guard has determined that with fresh water people can survive in a life raft 8 to 18 days without any food. The Coast Guard also believes you need a minimum of 800 calories a day for survival; but that sitting in a life raft, not being very active and just focused on pure survival. However, if you are in a situation where you're not moving and have to ration, use that 800 calories as a baseline.

# For Your Home

Once you go through your stockpile, what is left?

*Food expiration dates:*, There are several terms stamped on the food. This is what they mean:

SELL BY: How long a store should display the product for sale. This is a guide for the store. It is optimum quality date, but food is still edible for a while after.

BEST IF USED BY OR BEFORE DATE: This is only about quality, not safety.

GUARANTEED FRESH DATE: This usually refers to bakery items. They will still be edible after that date.

USE BY DATE: This is the last recommended day to use the product at peak quality. It is still edible after this.

PACK DATE: This is on canned and packaged goods. This actually might not be clear as sometimes its in code. It can be done by month-day-year as MMDDYY. Or it could be Julian calendar for the year, which means January is 001-0031. December would be 334-365.

Foods not to eat past their expiration date?

Eggs. Deli meat. Mixed greens. Alfalfa sprouts. Oysters. Shrimp. Raw ground beef. Berries. Soft cheese. Chicken.

So how long is food usually good for?

Milk: a week after Sell By.

Eggs: Three to five weeks after you buy them. Double-grade A will go down a grade in a week, but are still edible.

Poultry and seafood: Cook or freeze within a day.

Beef and pork: Cook or freeze within three to four days.

Canned good: High acid foods such as tomato sauce can last to 18 months. Low acid such as canned green beans can last for five years. However, do not store these in a hot space. A dry, cool place, is best.

*Grow a garden.* If you have the ground, plant the seeds at the appropriate time. This is a sustainable source of food. It is seasonal in most places, unless you have a greenhouse. However, it is also a fixed location.

# Food In Nature

Depending on your skills, your location and your needs, you might turn to food in nature before you turn to scavenging. We'll tackle some basic techniques here.

*Gathering*: cultivated plants, wild edible plants, insects, birds eggs.

*Hunting*: You need the means to hunt. Normally that means firearms, although skilled crossbow and bow hunters will be very valuable. Firearms have a noise signature. Arrows don't.

As far as field expedient weapons such as spears, bows, etc. that is beyond our scope here. Not only do you have to make them, you'd have to become proficient.

Hunting is recommended for large game, with a large return in terms of not only meat but other by-products.

If you have a .22 caliber rifle, the sound signature is much less, and you can carry many more rounds. But you will also be hunting much smaller game. Remember, though, that there is more small game than large game.

All mammals are edible and excellent protein sources (except the polar bear and bearded seal have toxin in the livers). Remember, though, that a wounded animal, even something as small as a raccoon, can cause nasty wounds which run the risk of infection.

Unless you are already a hunter, focus on . . .

*Trapping*: In your Grab-n-Go bag are ready made snares. Remember? Here they are in case you skipped the Prepare book:

Dakota Line Versatile Snares: http://amzn.to/2e2AuFv or their equivalent.

You might have wondered at the time why they were included. Now you know. While there are field expedient traps you can make, this is the simplest and most effective way.

Snares are very effective for harvesting small game. They were used by our ancient ancestors and they still work. The ones you have are lightweight, easy to pack and relatively easy to use.

Your snare is made from tightly wound steel cable five or more feet long. They have a one way locking mechanism on one end and a swivel and loop on the other.

First, find a trail where the game you're after is known to travel. Look for worn trails through the underbrush.

Anchor your snare. Use wire, such as from a coat hangar, slide it through the loop, and tie it around the base of a tree or post. Make sure the wire can't be pulled apart or unwound by the animal as it fights the trap.

Find a stick as the stand for the snare. Prop it up between the anchor point and the loop for snare. Have the slide lock of the loop about a half inch in front of the support. Essentially you're hanging a noose down over the trail. Once you're in place, push the stick down into the ground fixing it in place. The loop must be at the proper height for your target—where it's head would go into the loop. This is from 3 inches to 10 inches off the ground.

Set multiple snares to increase your odds. This is another way trapping is more effective than hunting.

Check your traps every day. The animal will be dead because the sliding lock closes around their necks and either cuts off circulation or breaks their neck during their initial struggle to get free.

Some notes on trapping:

Animals have to drink. Trails to watering holes are excellent places to emplace snares.

Don't disturb the area where you emplace your snare any more than necessary. Have all your parts ready, then go to the location and emplace. Do not use freshly cut vegetation in either the snare or to channel animals as the sap gives off an odor. Most mammals you are hunting depend heavily on their sense of smell for protection. You can use the fluid from the gall and urine bladders of previous kills to mask your scent. Coat your hands with it before assembling the snare. You can also 'smoke' the traps to remove your scent.

You can build a 'channel' along the trail to ensure the target runs into the snare, but the odds are doing so will leave too much odor and visual sign. However, few wild animals will back up.

You can bait a trap, but it must be a bait the target wants and isn't readily available all around. Peanut butter is a good bait. So is salt.

To field dress what you've caught:

First make sure it's really dead. Even the smallest critter can bite or claw you. Use a club.

Hang the animal by its back legs. Slice into the skin on both legs at the ankle. Pull down on the skin. It comes off like a glove. Remove the head and feet. Squirrels tend to be a bit tougher. Slice the skin on its back about two inches. Reach in, grasp both sides and pull them apart.

Gut it by pinching the upper stomach and make a small incision. Open the stomach cavity up and down. Remove the inner organs, being careful not to rupture the bladder. Keep the kidneys, heart and liver (you will use those in a stew).

Cook the meat.

This is very basic, but it will get you started and get you food.

*Fishing*: In your Grab-n-Go bag, you have some basic fishing essentials. Line, hooks. What is your experience level? Some basic guidelines on survival fishing:

Fish tend to feed before a storm, not after.

Light attracts fish at night.

Fish gather where there are deep pools, overhanging trees and brush, and around submerged foliage and logs that offer shelter.

There are no poisonous freshwater fish. Catfish do have needle-like protrusions on their dorsal fins that can inflict painful wounds, which leave you open to infection.

Cook all freshwater fish to kill parasites.

Cook saltwater fish caught inside of a reef or under the influence of a freshwater source. Fish caught in the sea can be eaten raw because of the salt water. However, there are some poisonous saltwater fish such as porcupine, triggerfish, cowfish, oilfish, thorn fish and red snapper.

How to do it:

Identify the best location.

Set multiple lines. Use trees branches hanging over the water instead of poles. Tie a baited hook, with a weight, on a line. For bait use live worms. Pretty much anything that crawls and you can put on the hook will serve. Once you start catching fish, use can use pieces of those fish as bait.

There are other living creatures that are edible. Frogs, snakes, etc. However, that's getting far into the survival mode.

*Plants*:

Think of two types of edible plants. Cultivated crops and certain plants in the wild.

When you did your Area Study, you noted what crops are grown in your locale. Which are edible? How do you make them edible? Some, such as corn, as obvious. Others require more study.

Edible plants have such a wide array across so many different climates and environs, there isn't the space to cover them here. Particularly to describe them.

A person who can recognize plants, which are edible, which are useful for other purposes such as herbs, and also grow them, is as valuable to a survival team than a top notch hunter.

It is much more likely that after you finish your stockpile of food you will turn to scavenging the man-made food supply.

## Scavenge

Reverse the food distribution network. The consumer gets food from a store. A store gets food delivered from a warehouse or a local producer. The warehouse gets food from where? Locally? Another distribution center? This goes on until we get to the true source of the food.

Where in that chain can you intervene and get food?

More on this under Scavenge, as food is just one many items you will be looking for.

## Sustain

*Grow a garden.* If you have the ground, plant the seeds at the appropriate time. This is a sustainable source of food. It is seasonal in most places, unless you have a greenhouse. However, it is also a fixed location. If you are enterprising, you could camouflage your garden out in nature, mixing up your edible plants in a forest or field, but be aware animals and birds like edible plants also.

*Be a hunter/gather* on the move.

*Barter*: Some skills will be worth others paying for in terms of food. Medical expertise is one such skill set.

More on this under Sustain.

# BUILDING A SHELTER AND STARTING A FIRE

As we discussed in Prepare, your home is your primary shelter. You've also designated an ERP that has a shelter nearby.

Beyond that, unless you're in the middle of nowhere, mankind has built millions of possible shelters, ranging from homes, factories, schools, churches, warehouses, etc.

If you aren't in your home, your Grab-n-Go bag has shelter, ranging from a tent, to a poncho, to an emergency sleeping bag.

A shelter is anything that can protect against not only the elements, but also danger. That means other people, but also the danger attendant with various emergencies and catastrophes.

In extreme emergencies, shelter can become the number one priority not only because we can survive only 3 hours with an un-regulated body temperature, but also because shelter can protect us against various other threats. So let's start with . . .

# Clothing

You're stuck with what you've prepared or what you're wearing. Here are key factors to keep in mind:

STAY DRY as much as possible.

Layer clothing in a cold weather environment.

Inner layer. Whatever is directly against your skin. The goal is to wick moisture away from your skin to the next two layers. Your body heat does the work, so the better the material for this, the less your body your body has to expend. This layer should have a snug fit around your body, as the body's heat is what wicks the moisture. The material used should absorb less than one percent of moisture.

Middle layer. This layer is your insulation. Its purpose is to keep your warmth, while it also helps wick away the moisture to the outer layer. This middle layer must move the moisture outward while keeping heat in. When you think middle layer, consider several garments instead of just one, so you can adjust as the temperature changes.

Outer layer. The primary purpose of the outer layer is to battle outside elements, primarily wind and wet. If you do not have this outer layer, you must build a shelter.

Focus on socks, gloves and hats. Dry and clean socks are important. You lose 40% of your heat through your head. Your hands are your most valuable tools. Protect them with gloves.

Protect yourself from the sun, even at the risk of being uncomfortable with long sleeves and pants. Wear a hat. Light colors reflect sunlight, black absorb. As already noted in *Prepare Now*, your clothing and shelter material should match the environment to encourage camouflage.

Sweating in a cold weather environment can be a killer as you are covering your body with moisture. Use your layers as a variable to avoid that.

# Emergency Shelters

A field expedient shelter out in nature takes several times longer to build than you think. Consider that in terms of the threat. If its dark, do you have a light source? Or is it better to keep moving to stay warm?

Location is the first consideration. If there isn't a man-made scavenge-able one available, is there a natural shelter? Tree well, where a tree has fallen and the roots have opened a large hole? Burned out log? Cave? Rock overhand? A log with a dry spot underneath?

Get out of the rain and the wind.

If a natural shelter isn't available, and you don't have one in hand such as a tent or poncho, the first option is a lean-to; if you can build a fire and have the materials to build a shelter.

You face a key decision if you are losing body temperature. Do you build the shelter first or the fire? If its raining and you know you can't get a fire going, then the shelter comes first. If the warmth of exertion from building the shelter won't stop the onset of hypothermia, then the fire first.

A tarp shelter is the most basic shelter. Using the poncho and paracord that should be in all your Grab-n-Go bags, or scavenged from your environment. A few keys apply when putting one together:

Look for natural or manmade surroundings that give you a good location and enhance the shelter. Incorporating a wall, a blown down trees, a large rock, etc. as part of the shelter is a good idea. Notice prevailing wind. Have your opening facing away.

One key to all emergency shelters: Smaller is better! First, a smaller shelter is easier to build, using less materials. Second, it will keep your body heat enclosed. Third, it is less noticeable (if that's one of your concerns).

There are five main areas to consider for an emergency shelter:

*Urban*: The most important aspect to consider here is other human beings. In an extreme emergency, survival is more important than etiquette and sometimes even law. When I lived in South Korea, when the alert siren went off, everyone was required to go indoors via the closest door to you. Didn't matter whose it was. They had to let you in. During a civil disturbance or a riot or extreme emergency, don't hesitate to knock on doors, whether it be homes or shops, to get out of danger.

There are dangers to watch out for besides unfriendly people. Downed power lines, broken water mains, unstable ruins.

Cities are three dimensional. Look up. Going to upper floors of buildings gives you the high ground and a more easily defended position. However, it also traps you. Cities have a veritable maze underneath them. Subway lines, sewers, communication tunnels, steam tunnels. No human being knows the exact extent of what is under New York City. Chicago has old coal tunnels that few people are aware of. These are things you looked for in your Area Study.

A key to remember with all emergency shelter in crowded areas is that others will also be seeking shelter.

*Forest*: The most desperate shelter is the debris hut. Just gather as much material around you as you can and bury yourself in it. If you have any sort of waterproof material put it as the outer layer, just like with clothing. Putting waterproof material next to your body traps your body's moisture and makes you wet.

Use as many branches and sticks to make a solid frame. Tie some together, or lacking paracord or other tying material, jam them into the ground and against each other. Then layer branches, leaves, sod, etcetera over the framework as tightly as possible without collapsing it.

*Jungle*: Essential the same as the debris hut, except you have more material to work with. You have vines, hollow shoots, larger leaves and the ground is usually softer and often provides clay. A key in the jungle shelter is get out of the moisture. In a swamp you want to put your shelter on the highest piece of ground you can find. Even a few inches can make a difference.

*Snow/Winter*: While survival shows have people building igloos and snow caves, these are time and labor intensive. Certainly, if you have both resources and time you can build them. However, my experience is that a snow trench is the simplest to build, if you have a poncho or other material to cover it. Once more, smaller is better. Dig a trench long enough and narrow enough for you to get into. Deep enough for you to be below the top surface of the snow. Make sure you put something at the bottom to keep your body off the snow. Put the poncho or tarp over the top, using snow to anchor each side. Leave a small opening you can slide in and out of and that you can fix in place.

A snow cave is similar except you are going deeper into the snow (thus requiring deeper snow) and leaving a snow roof in place. To fix the sides of a trench or cave, and the roof of a cave, use a candle or lighter to glaze the snow, briefly melting it, then allowing the temperature to turn it into ice.

*Desert*: Are you going to be traveling or not? If you're going to be moving you need a shelter for the day, to keep you as cool as possible and out of the sun, as you'll be traveling at night. If you're not traveling, then your shelter also has to work at night. As we noted discussing Desert survival, it often gets quite cold at night in the desert.

Use any vegetation available such as a juniper tree or sagebrush. Use piled up sand or rocks for one side of a shelter. If you can, dig into the ground. A belowground shelter can reduce the temperature thirty degrees. If necessary, use a layer of clothing as a block for the sun away from your body.

## Building a Fire

You have windproof lighters and matches in your Grab-n-Go bags. Even on your survival vest. Also a magnesium fire starter which you've practiced with.

Some caveats on fire starting. Make sure whatever you start doesn't get out of control. Fire is our friend until it becomes our enemy.

There are keys to starting any fire. First is gathering the proper flammables. They should be dry. If your environment is damp or wet, search for dry material under hanging rocks, under logs, or even gather damp material and put inside your shirt to use your body warmth to dry it out. Breaking damp sticks should expose a dry portion. Don't use soggy or rotten wood.

You need three piles:

Tinder: Dry, flammable material that needs only a few sparks to ignite. Thin, fibrous plant material. Fine steel wool. Tinder is easy to ignite but does not sustain fire. So you need . . .

Kindling: Slightly larger organic material that feeds the fire initially. Dry wood chips, twigs, dry strips of bark, dry grass stalks, refuse such as paper.

Firewood: Thicker branches and logs take longer to ignite, but once they do, they sustain the fire longer.

Field expedient ways:

Hand drill: The easiest field expedient way to build a fire is also the most labor intensive. Use a piece of hardwood as the fireboard. Make a notch in it with a knife or pointed rock. You need to a two-foot-long stick whose tip fits into the notch. Surround the notch with tinder. Roll the stick between your palms (wear gloves if you have them), causing friction. Enough friction causes heat. It will start smoking and ignite the kindling. Slowly add kindling.

Mirror/Glass: This requires two items. Sunlight and a parabolic mirror or lens. The reflector of a flashlight, the clean inside of a soda can are possibilities in a pinch. A clear bottle filled with water. Anything that can focus the rays of the sun.

Sustaining a long term fire: keep the flames going. If a fire burns down to embers, you use the core of that to restart the fire, using the same flow as starting a new fire: tinder, kindling, firewood. Tossing firewood on embers could disperse the embers and cause you to start over again.

# Emergency Rally Point/Base Camp

Your ERP is the alternative to your home. If you did not make it to your ERP or the ERP was not viable, you can establish a base camp that serves the same function.

It is where you plan to survive during a moderate to extreme emergency when your home is untenable.

When thinking about an ERP or base camp, use the term BLISS.

### BLISS considerations for the ERP
Blends in with surrounding
Low in silhouette
Irregular in shape
Small in size
Secluded

There are, of course, exception to this guideline. There might be a time when bunkering up in a high rise might be a good option. This is if a massive chemical/biological attack makes a top floor position desirable.

The key to the ERP/base camp is to stay hidden. That's your best defense. It is where you rest, recover, and live. How long depends on the emergency.

A key to the hide site is a Catch-22: water. You need water, yet water will draw predators, both human and otherwise. Consider locating the site about a half hour walk from a water source. That allows you to draw water, but not be so close that casual passerby's will stumble across your site.

The ERP/base camp should have concealment first and cover second. The difference between the two is this: concealment means you are hidden from observation. Cover means the position has protection against direct and indirect fire weapons (remember, arrows are indirect fire, as Custer learned). The reason I prioritize concealment over cover is because the best defense is not to be found.

How do you get to your ERP? If you drive to it, make sure to leave the vehicle far enough away, at least two miles, so that it doesn't point others toward your site. Disable the vehicles by taking an engine part. Assume the vehicle will be looted, but perhaps you can use it if you return with the part. The easiest part to take is the main fuse. You can conceal the vehicle as much as possible, but if you drove it there, it's on a trail that takes vehicles which means others can drive there too.

Another thing to consider is putting your site behind a gate that can be locked. Many parks, logging roads, etc, have lockable gates. Cut the current lock on it, drive through, out of sight, and put your own lock on the gate. Still, keep at least a two mile distance between the vehicle and your hide site.

As soon as you are settled in your site, search out an escape route and a Rally Point and make sure everyone knows where it is. The Rally Point is where you will all meet if the site is attacked.

When getting water, don't use the same trail all the time. Mix it up.

Always maintain security. One person must be up and alert at all times.

# Should I Stay or Should I Keep On The Move?

There are too many variables to be able to make this decision until you are actually in the situation. The most important is what is the nature of the emergency or catastrophe?

Is your ERP/base camp under threat?

In extreme emergencies, more and more people will be moving out of urban areas. What was secure at the beginning of the emergency might become insecure later on.

Are you running out of scavenging supplies if you've reached that phase? Remember, though, that scavenging is taking place everywhere. Just moving might not improve the situation. It might be better to stay and move to sustainment.

You should always *be prepared to move*. This means keeping your Grab-n-Go bag packed as much as possible. Don't leave your gear strewn about everywhere. Be able to tear down your tent or tarp quickly and stuff it in the bag.

There are dangers to being on the move. You could run into strangers who are not friendly or desire to scavenge off of you.

Do you have a destination? Just moving with no destination is demoralizing and serves little purpose.

# Scavenge

Scavenging shelter means occupying buildings or facilities that provide shelter. Or scouring what's available for material with which to build an expedient shelter.

More on this in the Scavenge Section.

# Sustain

Water is the priority. Next is food. Can you build a sustainable site?

More on this in the Sustain Section.

# NAVIGATING, TRACKING

In an emergency situation, especially moderate to extreme, it is highly possible you will have to move from point A to point B. It is likely you won't have a GPS to do that with.

So let's walk through basic land navigation before briefly touching on tracking and evasion.

Based on Prepare Now, you've already downloaded or purchased topographic maps.

Your map is a very valuable document. Treat is as one. Keep it in the waterproof map case you have and keep it tied off to your body.

When you look at a topo map, you immediately see that it's different than your road map. Features on it include:

Roads, buildings, boundaries, railways, power transmission lines. Etc. In Germany, the maps were so accurate that actually had fence lines around fields on them.

Water: lakes, rivers, streams, swamps, rapids, kraken, etc.

Relief: mountains, valleys, slopes, depressions, ridges, knolls, gnomes, etc.

Vegetation: forested or clear areas, orchards, vineyards, Ents, etc.

Toponymy: a fancy word for the names of the various things on the map.

Use the map legend to learn how to use the symbols, colors and lines on the map.

Scale is the relationship between size on the map and in the real world. One thing I've noted on many GPS systems is that they don't indicate scale since they give directions and distance. This can be disorienting. Everything always looks a lot closer on a map than when you're walking.

**Legend**

It gives you a guide to the various symbols on the map. The types of roads will be defined in the Legend.

**Contour lines**

This gives you an idea if elevation. If you trace a contour line on the map, you are tracing a line of equal elevation. If you walked that line, you will not go up or down. Check the legend for the contour interval—this is critical. There's a big difference between a 10 meter contour interval and a 50 meter one. As you go from one contour line to the next, that is the contour interval difference. Usually contour interval is based on the terrain the map covers. Relatively flat terrain will have very short interval, while mountainous terrain might intervals as great as 100 meters. Every fifth contour line is an index and labeled with a number.

The closer lines are, the steeper the terrain. When they're piled on top of each other, that means a cliff. Do not walk off it. If they are very far apart, that equals relatively smooth terrain. Notice how counter lines always dive in toward streams and rivers.

The key to using a map is orienting it to the terrain. While there are many field-expedient ways of doing this, the easiest is to orient using a compass. Next easiest is to use roads or easily identifiable terrain features around you.

But suppose you don't have a compass or readily identifiable terrain features?

**Using the sun and shadows**

The earth's relationship to the sun can help you to determine direction. The sun rises in the east and sets in the west, but not exactly due east or due west. There is also some seasonal variation. In the northern hemisphere, the sun will be due south when at its highest point in the sky, or when an object casts no appreciable shadow. In the southern hemisphere, this same noon day sun will mark due north. In the northern hemisphere, shadows will move clockwise. Shadows will move counterclockwise in the southern hemisphere.

The shadow methods used for direction finding are the shadow-tip and watch methods.

### Shadow-Tip Method

Find a straight stick 3 feet long and an open, level spot on which the stick will cast a definite shadow.

*Step 1.* Place the stick or branch into the ground where it will cast a distinctive shadow. Mark the shadow's tip. This first shadow mark is always west —**everywhere** on earth.

*Step 2.* Wait until the shadow tip moves a few inches. Mark the shadow tip's new position.

*Step 3.* Draw a straight line through the two marks to obtain an approximate east-west line.

*Step 4.* Stand with the first mark (west) to your left and the second mark to your right-you are now facing north. This fact is true **everywhere** on earth.

### The Watch Method

You can also determine direction using a common or analog watch—one that has hands. The direction will be accurate if you are using true local time, without any changes for daylight savings time. Remember, the further you are from the equator, the more accurate this method will be. If you only have a digital watch, you can overcome this obstacle. Quickly draw a watch on a circle of paper with the correct time on it and use it to determine your direction at that time.

105

In the northern hemisphere, hold the watch horizontal and point the hour hand at the sun. Bisect the angle between the hour hand and the 12 o'clock mark to get the north-south line (Figure 18-2). If there is any doubt as to which end of the line is north, remember that the sun rises in the east, sets in the west, and is due south at noon. The sun is in the east before noon and in the west after noon.

Note: If your watch is set on daylight savings time, use the midway point between the hour hand and 1 o'clock to determine the north-south line.

In the southern hemisphere, point the watch's 12 o'clock mark toward the sun and a midpoint halfway between 12 and the hour hand will give you the north-south line.

### Using the Moon

Because the moon has no light of its own, we can only see it when it reflects the sun's light. As it orbits the earth on its 28-day circuit, the shape of the reflected light varies according to its position. We say there is a new moon or no moon when it is on the opposite side of the earth from the sun. Then, as it moves away from the earth's shadow, it begins to reflect light from its right side and waxes to become a full moon before waning, or losing shape, to appear as a sliver on the left side. You can use this information to identify direction.

If the moon rises before the sun has set, the illuminated side will be the west. If the moon rises after midnight, the illuminated side will be the east. This obvious discovery provides us with a rough east-west reference during the night.

### Using the Stars

Your location in the Northern or Southern Hemisphere determines which constellation you use to determine your north or south direction.

### The Northern Sky

The main constellations to learn are the Ursa Major, also known as the Big Dipper or the Plow, and Cassiopeia (Figure 18-3). Neither of these constellations ever sets. They are always visible on a clear night. Use them to locate Polaris, also known as the polestar or the North Star. The North Star forms part of the Little Dipper handle and can be confused with the Big Dipper. Prevent confusion by using both the Big Dipper and Cassiopeia together. The Big Dipper and Cassiopeia are always directly opposite each other and rotate counterclockwise around Polaris, with Polaris in the center. The Big Dipper is a seven star constellation in the shape of a dipper. The two stars forming the outer lip of this dipper are the "pointer stars" because they point to the North Star. Mentally draw a line from the outer bottom star to the outer top star of the Big Dipper's bucket. Extend this line about five times the distance between the pointer stars. You will find the North Star along this line.

Cassiopeia has five stars that form a shape like a "W" on its side. The North Star is straight out from Cassiopeia's center star. After locating the North Star, locate the North Pole or true north by drawing an imaginary line directly to the earth.

BOB MAYER

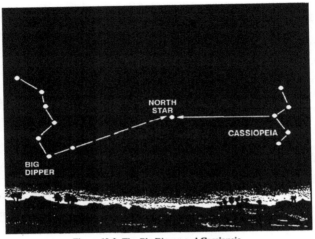

**Figure 18-3. The Big Dipper and Cassiopeia.**

## The Southern Sky

Because there is no star bright enough to be easily recognized near the south celestial pole, a constellation known as the Southern Cross is used as a sign post to the South (Figure18-4).

The Southern Crossor Crux hasfivestars. Its four brightest stars form a cross that tilts to one side. The two stars that make up the cross's long axis are the pointer stars. To determine south, imagine a distance five times the distance between These stars and the point where this imaginary line ends is in the general direction of south. Look down to the horizon from this imaginary point and select a landmark to steerby. In a static survival situation you can fix this location in daylight if you drive stakes in the ground at night to point the way.

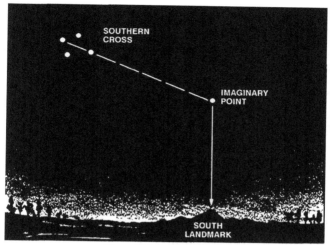

Figure 18-4. Southern Cross.

### Navigation.

Water flows downhill. That sounds basics, but sometimes we need to remind ourselves of the basics.

You've covered this already in your Area Study, but to update. Know which side of the Continental Divide or the Appalachians you are on. The Rockies and the Appalachian Mountains have divides. Study a map of your region. What are the major streams and rivers? Where do they join? How many bridges cross them? Where? Remember, bridges are chokepoints.

Are there any significant terrain features in your area that are noticeable from a distance? Pilots Peak in Utah was a landmark for many people traveling west.

Know your pace count. This is how many times your right foot hits the ground per one hundred meters. This allows you to stay oriented. You can go to the local high school and pace off one hundred yards, which is close to one hundred meters (a yard is slightly longer). But remember, that will be on flat ground. Pace count changes greatly when you move through rough terrain.

### Tracking and Evasion

This usually comes into play during an extreme emergency when there is conflict among peoplet. In order to understand how to evade being tracked down, you need to first understand how to track someone.

The key to tracking someone is not examining bent twigs, or marks in the dirt, but rather understanding the mindset and habits of whatever you are tracking. Predators tend to cluster near water sources in areas where water is scarce. Rather than tracking down their prey, they let their prey come to them. People tend to take the easiest path. That's why ambushes are set up along paths and choke points.

Where will whoever or whatever you are tracking be going? What is their destination? If you're very sure of their destination, perhaps you can get there before them. Will they need food? Water? When setting your snares for food, this is a key consideration.

To evade someone tracking you, you must avoid the easy way. You must break bad habits. You must confuse them. You must make it difficult for them to follow.

My first platoon sergeant told me an interesting thing: few people ever look up. Remember in *Hunger Games* when the heroine hides up in a tree? Like everything else, this is a double-edged thing: you might not be noticed, but if you are, as she was, you are trapped.

One of the best ways to avoid being followed is to use water. Few people want to wade through water or go into that swamp. A little discomfort can be worth your life.

Here are keys to evasion:

If ever captured, try to escape quickly. The longer you remain a prisoner, the lower your chances of escape.

If ever arrested, say nothing. You have the right to remain silent, then remain silent.

Don't be noticeable. Ever watch a crowd? Ever see the people who stand out? You don't want to be that person. A rule of survival on the New York subway is to not make eye contact. One of my rules is to never poke the crazy person. When walking down the street, avoid eye contact and all contact with those who could possibly be threats. When avoiding a riot or civil unrest, the same applies.

If your team has to evade, you must make an important decision: whether to break the group up into pairs or try to evade as a team. Remember, of course, that you are evading to a point, usually your ERP. So if any team members are captured, you must assume they will give up the location of the ERP. On the other hand, pairs have a greater chance of evasion than a large group.

Don't leave tracks. This seems obvious, but few of us have ever thought about it. And even fewer have ever looked behind ourselves to see if we are leaving tracks.

**In Conclusion**

The odds that you will have to track or evade are low in a mild or moderate emergency. But the odds you will have to land navigate without electronic aid isn't so low. Make sure you have maps, both road and topographical. Make sure you have a basic understanding of the terrain around you. Practice your routes from your home to you IRP and ERP and on to the Hide Site.

When traveling, plan your route and plan alternate routes.

# SPECIFIC ENVIRONMENTS AND EVENTS

You did an Area Study and have prepared for your environment and these possible events. Here are things to do.

## Your Survival Team

If you are not with your team, you are in the dangerous situation of considering whether to make it on your own or join forces. There are advantages and disadvantages to a team.

### Advantages

The whole is greater than the sum of its parts. You can't be an expert on everything. Having an array of people who bring different, needed skills, is important.

Some people just can't handle being alone. Can you?

A sense of purpose. In combat, soldiers fight for each other, not for a cause. Being a member of a team can increase your motivation to get out of yourself and fight for the survival of those who you care about and are with you.

In an extreme emergency, long term survival will eventually depend on team building. In this scenario you often won't have much of a choice who you will ally with.

Groups will form with different agendas. You have to evaluate your goals, and also whether you will be an asset to the team and whether the team will view you as an asset. What do you bring to the table?

### Disadvantages

You make a larger target. It is indeed better to run away rather than fight. Your running away is limited by your slowest member.

How prepared are the others?

Will the members of the team actually pull their weight?

### Team Building

The whole can be greater than the sum of the parts. Think what this means for survival. Honesty is the cornerstone of strong teamwork because it builds trust and respect. Do you trust with your life? And remember, the worse the emergency, the more people will lie, cheat and steal, and eventually, kill, placing their survival ahead of yours. There will also be those who won't. There are those who would give you the shirt off their back and those who would steal the shirt off your back.

A key decision that has to be made is a chain of command. Someone must be the leader.

A survival group is not a democracy. Often there is no time to sit around and debate options. Decisions have to be made quickly. Hammer out the leadership issue before the emergency.

### Team Communication

The first issue is going to be communicating. We are overly reliant on cell phone communication. In a moderate or extreme emergency, it is likely that this service will either be interrupted (lack of power, towers destroyed) or overwhelmed with too many people trying to call at the same time. On 9-11, many people were frustrated in their attempts to use their cell phones.

Also, if there is an extended power outage, even if service isn't interrupted, are you able to recharge your cell phone?

Texting has a higher likelihood of getting through than voice, so consider that if you are unable to get a call through during an emergency.

When you consider using a GPS on your cell phone, remember that in most cases, the mapping information is being downloaded from your net.

**Organizing Your Neighborhood/Work Place**

This is particularly key in moderate emergencies. During natural disasters such as hurricane, flood, extreme weather, wild fire, etc. an organized neighborhood can be essential to survival. When I say neighborhood, I also mean your work place.

Check out the resources in your neighborhood. Do you know who your neighbors are and what they do for a living? What special skills they have? That person you think is a nurse going off to work in her scrubs might actually be someone who works at a kennel washing dogs. Don't make assumptions.

*You need to identify people who have the following skills and experience:*

Medical
Law enforcement and military
Electrical
Leadership
Survival
Child care
Communications
Engineering
Weapons
Gardening

*Inventory equipment in the neighborhood:*
Chain saws
Winches
Four wheel drive vehicles
CB and other radios
Water purifying systems

*Inventory the neighborhood:*
Where are all the natural gas meters and propane tanks?
Who needs special help? Focus on the handicapped, the elderly, and children who might be home alone at periods of the day.

Each household should have large placards made up with OKAY on one side and HELP on the other. Use fluorescent colored poster board available at your local supermarket. Have this stored near a front window under a rug. Display as needed.

Determine where the neighborhood gathering site will be. People should go here before trying to run around and rescue others. Organization saves time and lives.

Have a contact tree of who alerts who. In the military we always had alert systems. This is a way of communicating so each person knows who they are responsible for contacting.

Since you've done your Area Study, you have a good idea of what you are facing in your area of operations.

Depending on where you live or travel, you must make special arrangements for extremes in terrain and weather. I'm going to briefly cover key points in preparing for four special environments: cold weather, desert, tropical and water survival.

# Cold Weather

1) Everything takes at least twice as long to achieve in cold weather.

2) Fire is eventually an essential. Whether for melting snow and ice into water, cooking meals, drying out clothing and gear, or just warming people up.

3) Moving on snow with equipment is extraordinarily hard.

4) Cold weather affects equipment in different ways. One key to remember is that any exposed water container will freeze. We quickly learned to keep our water source inside our clothing, allowing our body to keep it from freezing. The same with thawing out our next meal. On the positive side batteries keep their charge longer in the cold; in the bad side, they expand power faster when used.

Windchill is the effect of moving air on exposed flesh. Wind always exacerbates the situation, which is why your outer garment should not only be water resistant, but wind resistant. A key in building shelter is to get out of the wind.

Here is a handy chart showing the effect of wind chill.

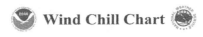

## Wind Chill Chart

| | Temperature (°F) | | | | | | | | | | | | | | | | | |
|---|---|---|---|---|---|---|---|---|---|---|---|---|---|---|---|---|---|---|
| Calm | 40 | 35 | 30 | 25 | 20 | 15 | 10 | 5 | 0 | -5 | -10 | -15 | -20 | -25 | -30 | -35 | -40 | -45 |
| 5 | 36 | 31 | 25 | 19 | 13 | 7 | 1 | -5 | -11 | -16 | -22 | -28 | -34 | -40 | -46 | -52 | -57 | -63 |
| 10 | 34 | 27 | 21 | 15 | 9 | 3 | -4 | -10 | -16 | -22 | -28 | -35 | -41 | -47 | -53 | -59 | -66 | -72 |
| 15 | 32 | 25 | 19 | 13 | 6 | 0 | -7 | -13 | -19 | -26 | -32 | -39 | -45 | -51 | -58 | -64 | -71 | -77 |
| 20 | 30 | 24 | 17 | 11 | 4 | -2 | -9 | -15 | -22 | -29 | -35 | -42 | -48 | -55 | -61 | -68 | -74 | -81 |
| 25 | 29 | 23 | 16 | 9 | 3 | -4 | -11 | -17 | -24 | -31 | -37 | -44 | -51 | -58 | -64 | -71 | -78 | -84 |
| 30 | 28 | 22 | 15 | 8 | 1 | -5 | -12 | -19 | -26 | -33 | -39 | -46 | -53 | -60 | -67 | -73 | -80 | -87 |
| 35 | 28 | 21 | 14 | 7 | 0 | -7 | -14 | -21 | -27 | -34 | -41 | -48 | -55 | -62 | -69 | -76 | -82 | -89 |
| 40 | 27 | 20 | 13 | 6 | -1 | -8 | -15 | -22 | -29 | -36 | -43 | -50 | -57 | -64 | -71 | -78 | -84 | -91 |
| 45 | 26 | 19 | 12 | 5 | -2 | -9 | -16 | -23 | -30 | -37 | -44 | -51 | -58 | -65 | -72 | -79 | -86 | -93 |
| 50 | 26 | 19 | 12 | 4 | -3 | -10 | -17 | -24 | -31 | -38 | -45 | -52 | -60 | -67 | -74 | -81 | -88 | -95 |
| 55 | 25 | 18 | 11 | 4 | -3 | -11 | -18 | -25 | -32 | -39 | -46 | -54 | -61 | -68 | -75 | -82 | -89 | -97 |
| 60 | 25 | 17 | 10 | 3 | -4 | -11 | -19 | -26 | -33 | -40 | -48 | -55 | -62 | -69 | -76 | -84 | -91 | -98 |

Frostbite Times  ▢ 30 minutes  ▢ 10 minutes  ▢ 5 minutes

Wind Chill (°F) = $35.74 + 0.6215T - 35.75(V^{0.16}) + 0.4275T(V^{0.16})$

Where, T= Air Temperature (°F)  V= Wind Speed (mph)  *Effective 11/01/01*

Always keep your head covered. You lose 40 to 45 percent of body heat from an unprotected head and even more from the unprotected neck, wrist, and ankles. These areas of the body are good radiators of heat and have very little insulating fat. The brain is very susceptible to cold and can stand the least amount of cooling. Because there is much blood circulation in the head, most of which is on the surface, you can lose heat quickly if you do not cover your head. This is also why scalp wounds tend to bleed profusely.

There are four basic principles to follow to keep warm. An easy way to remember these basic principles is to use the word COLD—

**C** keep clothing *Clean.*

**O** avoid *Overheating. (once more: sweating is very dangerous in the cold)*

**L** wear clothes *Loose* and in *Layers.*

**D** keep clothing *Dry.*

*C **Keep clothing clean.*** This principle is always important for sanitation and comfort. In winter, it is also important from the standpoint of warmth. Clothes matted with dirt and grease lose much of their insulation value. Heat can escape more easily from the body through the clothing's crushed or filled up air pockets.

*O **Avoid overheating.*** When you get too hot, you sweat and your clothing absorbs the moisture. This affects your warmth in two ways: dampness decreases the insulation quality of clothing, and as sweat evaporates, your body cools. Adjust your clothing so that you do not sweat. Do this by partially opening your parka or jacket, by removing an inner layer of clothing, by removing heavy outer mittens, or by throwing back your parka hood or changing to lighter headgear. The head and hands act as efficient heat dissipaters when overheated.

*L **Wear your clothing loose and in layers.*** Wearing tight clothing and footwear restricts blood circulation and invites cold injury. It also decreases the volume of air

117

trapped between the layers, reducing its insulating value. Several layers of lightweight clothing are better than one equally thick layer of clothing, because the layers have dead-air space between them. The dead-air space provides extra insulation. Also, layers of clothing allow you to take off or add clothing layers to prevent excessive sweating or to increase warmth.

*D Keep clothing dry.* In cold temperatures, your inner layers of clothing can become wet from sweat and your outer layer, if not water repellent, can become wet from snow and frost melted by body heat. Wear water repellent outer clothing, if available. It will shed most of the water collected from melting snow and frost. Before entering a heated shelter, brush off the snow and frost. Despite the precautions you take, there will be times when you cannot keep from getting wet. At such times, drying your clothing may become a major problem. On the march, hang your damp mittens and socks on your rucksack. Sometimes in freezing temperatures, the wind and sun will dry this clothing. You can also place damp socks or mittens, unfolded, near your body so that your body heat can dry them. In a campsite, hang damp clothing inside the shelter near the top, using drying lines or improvised racks. You may even be able to dry each item by holding it before an open fire. Dry leather items slowly. If no other means are available for drying your boots, put them between your sleeping bag shell and liner. Your body heat will help to dry the leather.

### Dehydration

When bundled up in many layers of clothing during cold weather, you may be unaware that you are losing body moisture. Your heavy clothing absorbs the moisture that normally evaporates in the air. You must drink water to replace this loss of fluid. Your need for water is as great in a cold environment as it is in a warm environment even though you don't feel as thirsty. In fact, we often don't want to drink water when we're cold.

One way to tell if you are becoming dehydrated is to check the color of your urine on snow. If your urine makes the snow dark yellow, you are becoming dehydrated and you need to replace body fluids. If it makes the snow light yellow to no color, your body fluids have a more normal balance. You can also smell the sharp odor of the urine when someone is dehydrated. It's very hard to make people drink water in a cold environment, which makes dehydration a particular danger. A team leader must keep track to make sure every person stays hydrated.

# Desert

*Intense sunlight and heat* are present in all arid areas. Air temperature can go well over 100 degrees F every day. The highest recorded temperature in the United States was 134 F in Death Valley. Heat comes from more than direct sunlight. Hot wind, reflective heat (sun bouncing off the sand/ground/rocks) and conductive heat when you make direct contact with the ground.

The ground is going to be much hotter than the air. For example, if the air is 110 F, the ground could easily be 140 F.

Naturally, your requirements for water will be much higher in a desert environment. Shelter is also as critical in this environment as in a cold weather environment. If you have to move, travel at night to avoid the sun. Equipment behaves differently under extreme temperatures. High temperatures affect batteries adversely and they will not last as long as usual.

*Wide Temperature Range:* Temperatures will vary widely in desert areas, particularly high desert. During the day it can be well over 100 F and at night quickly drop to below 50 F. This means you have to be prepared for both extremes, especially with clothing.

*Sparse Vegetation:* There is little vegetation in a desert area. This means you'll have a tougher time making an expedient shelter. Sometimes the best shelter you can find during the day is in the shadows. The temperature in a shaded area is significantly less than in the open. Also, reflective and conductive heat will be much less.

Another problem in the desert is estimating distance. On average, we underestimate distance by a factor of three. What looks like a mile away, is actually three miles away.

*Water requirements:* Your body sheds heat by sweating. The hotter you are, the more you sweat. While in a cold weather environment you can modulate this by shedding layers of clothing, in a desert you don't have this option. What you can do is conserve your sweat as much as possible. Wear clothing that covers you. This not only protects you from the sun, and the wind heat, but it absorbs your sweat and keeps it next to your body as long as possible rather than getting immediately evaporated.

Limit eating as much as possible. Food requires water for digestion, so you are walking a fine line. Remember that water is more vital than food.

You cannot trust your sense of thirst to determine your water requirement. It's been found that a person who relies on thirst drinks only two-thirds of what they actually require.

# Tropical

A tropical region has high temperatures, heavy rainfall, and high humidity. Tropics cover about seven percent of the world's land surface but contain over fifty percent of the species. Temperatures rarely fall before freezing, unless one is at altitude.

Since the tropics are near the equator, day and night are usually of roughly equal length. Night tends to come quickly, as does dawn.

On the plus side, the tropical environment provides plenty of raw material for shelter, food and water is plentiful. On the negative side, germs and parasites multiply at an alarming rate.

# Specific Man-Made Events— Transportation

### Car

*Tornados*. If you can see a tornado, drive away from it as quickly and safely as possible. Move at right angles to the tornado. If you can, stop and seek shelter in a building or underground, such as a culvert. If you get caught while in the car, do NOT get out of the car. It's not entirely safe, but it's better than the options. Pull off the road, out of traffic, because that other idiot is still going to be barreling down the road at 70 miles an hour even though he can't see. Make sure you have your set belt on. Put your head down to avoid broken glass and hurled objects. Cover your head with a blanket or jacket. Do NOT seek shelter under overpasses. Tornados can move at sixty miles an hour, so think hard before trying to out-run one. To get an idea of the path of the storm, pick a stationery object near you and watch how the tornado moves in relation to that object. If it is moving to your left, drive to the right and vice versa. If it doesn't seem to be moving left or right, then it's either coming right at you or away from you. If it's getting bigger, guess which of the two? Get out of the car and seek safety in a building or culvert if you have the time.

*Fire*: If you smell burning rubber or plastic or any smoke, immediately pull over to a safe place and check it out. If a fuse continues to go out, that's a sign of a short.

Don't ignore it. Get the car checked out. You must carry a fire extinguisher in your vehicle, if the fire is fueled by your gas line, forget about using it and get a safe distance away. At least 150 feet. Warn others in the area and keep them away while calling 911.

If you skid, turn into the skid to straighten out.

Never, ever, use gas to start a fire.

## Plane Crash

Where to sit? Statistics from crashes indicate it's safest to sit in the rear of the plane. Yes, I know it takes longer to get on and off, but that's what the numbers show. Despite that, I prefer to be near an exit. I'll take the exit row every time, and not just for the extra room.

What to wear? There is a reason military flight crews wear a specific outfit. It's because the greatest danger is flame. Wear long pants, a long sleeve shirt, and shoes you can move quickly in: ie, don't be doing the Hawaiian shirt, shorts and sandals.

Keep your seat belt fastened at all times. Flight attendants will tell you horror stories of abrupt, unexpected turbulence that bounced them off the ceiling of the plane.

Brace for impact. Feet flat on floor, head tucked in.

If the oxygen masks drop, do put yours on before helping others.

What is the most important thing to know? Where the closest exit is. Yes, turn and look behind you. Orient yourself to the plane. They put that safety lighting along the aisles in after learning that in the smoke and confusion of a crash, people quickly became disoriented.

When evacuating the plane, get away from it. At least five hundred feet upwind of the plane. Burning fuel is the most dangerous element after a crash.

Yes, when evacuating, leave it all behind. That computer is not worth your life or the lives of others.

If you have to put on your life vest (yes, you're screwed), DO NOT inflate it until you are out of the plane. Inflating it inside and then having a water landing, simply traps you inside the plane as the water pouring in will pin you against whatever part of the plane is right side up.

If your plane crashes in a remote area, should you stay with the plane or not? Stay. Most planes have a transponder. And it's easier to find a crash site than you wandering in the wilderness.

Shift into scavenge mode, using the plane as the source.

## Specific Man-Made Events—Safety and Security

### Power Outage

Cook perishable foods first. Of course, you can only do that if you have that secondary cooking source, which was covered under equipment. Do NOT use gas grills or stoves inside. They release carbon monoxide and can cause death.

Do you have a back up method for heating and cooling? For heating, a fireplace works. If you have propane in a tank, can you start your fireplace or heating systems without electricity? Do you know how to work the pilot light and clicker? For cooling, there are portable fans that are battery powered, but they have limited life. Have you considered getting a generator? That house that I just purchased has a whole house generator that kicks in automatically when the power goes out. It's claimed that it can power the entire house for a week on one tank of propane. However, the reality is, if you use a generator, cut power outage down to the absolutely essential: refrigerator and heating and cooling at the margins. Turn off all unnecessary power users. It is *not* business as usual.

Use your crank power radio for the latest news.

Close the curtains to keep heat or cool in. Also, remember, a basement will be the most consistent in terms of temperature.

123

### Fire

If your clothes catch on fire, Stop-Drop-Roll, to put the fire out.

Close doors behind you as you leave.

If you touch a door handle and its hot, or the door itself is hot, don't open that door.

Once out, do not go back in.

If you're trapped inside the house, stay in a room with the doors closed. Place a wet towel under the door opening and call 911. If you have a window, open it and wave something colorful or use a flashlight at night.

If you have to escape through smoke, go low, under the smoke.

If you use a fire extinguisher remember the acronym PASS:

Pull the pin and hold the extinguisher facing away from you.

Aim low. Point the extinguisher at the base of the fire.

Squeeze the handle.

Sweep the extinguisher from side to side until the fire is out.

### Robbery

This is when you are confronted outside of your home and someone wants to take something of value from you, whether it be your wallet, purse, watch, car, etc.

The rule is simple: give it up.

You are more valuable than any material object.

The most important thing is to remain calm and don't panic. Remember, the robber is often in a turbulent emotional state and could be under the influence of drugs or alcohol. Your panic could add to their panic.

Make eye contact while you agree to comply. Move slowly. Hand over whatever they want. Do not act overly weak or aggressive. Try to remember as much about them as possible. Let them get away, then call 911.

### Civil Unrest and Riots

This can quickly become an extreme emergency on a local or large-scale level. The psychology of crowds is very interesting, but suffice it to say people act very differently when in groups and especially when scared and/or angry.

To get through the initial stages of a riot, you must learn how to survive your fellow human beings.

If you can prepare and have to travel through an area that might have a riot, carry a solution for rinsing your eyes out in case of tear gas.

Make sure you have identification.

When traveling, aim for as many crossroads as possible because they give you three options for directions.

Remain calm.

Hide. Avoidance is always best.

Blend in while moving away. Avoid law enforcement if they have donned their riot gear because they will tend to arrest first and ask questions later.

If you must pass through rioters/looters/etc. wear long sleeves, long pants, consider a motorcycle or other helmet.

Walk, don't run. Don't make eye contact. Don't confront people. Don't stop. Don't run as you might attract attention. If you're with someone from your team, hold hands tightly.

Don't get involved. It's not your riot.

Stay close to walls, on the edges of crowds. Avoid bottlenecks.

If you're in your car, don't stop. You are in a position of power as long you keep moving, slowly but surely. Don't speed up or act aggressive. People will give way. Keep your doors locked and your windows up.

Riots usually happen on streets, not in buildings. Get off the street and into a building. Stay away from windows. Look for another exit. Be careful of fire.

If necessary, on foot, go with the flow. Become part of the crowd and edge your path away from the violence.

### Terrorist Attack

Top targets for homicide bombers: subways, train and busses. Malls. Restaurants and night clubs. Stadiums. Movie theaters. Schools. Churches. In essence, places where people gather together tightly. Whenever you are in such a place, you should always be aware of where the nearest exit is. Actually, any time you're indoors, you should always know where the exits are. That knowledge can save your life. Think if the power goes off, a fire starts, someone begins shooting. In the panic, it's hard to do what you should have done upon first entering the place.

Be aware. Those warnings not to leave your luggage unattended in the airport are serious. If you see someone walk away from a bag, that's something you shouldn't ignore.

If you are ever in a hostage situation, realize that when the good guys break in to free you, they're going to cuff everyone until they can sort out who is who. A trick kidnappers can play is to tape toy guns to hostages' hands, or pretend to be hostages themselves in order to escape. Let the experts do their job.

If you are at home and hear of a terrorist attack nearby, stay at home. Do not go out. Listen to reliable media sources.

A homicide bomber is carrying a bomb. That sounds self-explanatory, but you need to consider where the bomb is. If it's a vest, they will appear unnaturally bulky. If someone is wearing a coat or jacket that is inappropriate to the weather, that's a warning sign. If they're carrying it in a backpack, briefcase, etc. they often will clutch it to their chest just prior to detonation.

If a bomb goes off, be aware that a common plot is to have follow on bombs designated to kill the first responders. Do not gather in the area unless you are helping those injured, and even then, be aware there could be secondary or follow on attacks.

While it is best to run away, as a last ditch effort, an effective way to disrupt a homicide bomber is to go low and take their legs out from under them. It is an instinct that a person will put out their hands to break their fall, thus releasing the detonation switch. Unless it's a dead man's switch in which case releasing it makes it go off. It's pretty much a sucky situation all around and you can only do the best you can.

**Active Shooter**
Remember these three words: RUN. HIDE. FIGHT.

If you can, evacuate. Leave regardless of what others want to do. Leave everything behind, just like escaping a plane. Help others escape if they want to come, but do not move wounded people. Keep your hands visible as you exit so police can see you are not armed. Follow the instructions of the police, no matter what they tell you to do. If they tell you face down on the ground, get face down on the ground. There is a good chance you will be cuffed.

If you can't evacuate. If you are in a hallway, get into the nearest room.

Secure the door in the room. Lock it and blockade it with the heaviest objects you can place against it. Silence your cell phone. Turn off any other sources of noise. Hide behind large objects (desks, filing cabinets, etc.).

Remain quiet.

Call 911. If you can't talk, leave the phone on so the dispatcher can listen.

If, as a last resort, you must take action, act aggressively and without reserve. Throw whatever is handy, scream and charge. Take them down.

Understand how law enforcement will be reacting.

They will usually assault in teams. They could be wearing a variety of uniforms, since they might be responding from different agencies. They might use gas, flash-bangs, and other non-lethals to secure an area.

Do not have anything in your hands. Keep your hands visible at all times. Don't make any quick movements. If they are passing you by, searching for the shooter, move in the direction they came from. Remember, the initial breaching team will not stop to provide assistance to wounded. They are going for the shooter. Medical personnel will be following. If you are able, help the medical personnel as they arrive.

If you can, provide police or the dispatcher with the following information:

Location of the shooter. Number of shooters. Description of shooter. Number and type of weapons. Number and location of victims.

Once you are out, you will be held in an area until the situation is under control. Do not leave until instructed.


## Specific Man-Made Events—Nuclear, Biological and Chemical

### Nuclear Plants
Here are the keys to minimize your exposure:

Distance. Get away. The further you are from the source of the radiation, the better. If it is going into the air, check prevailing wind patterns. If you want some history on this, check out how Chernobyl dispersed radiation across Russia and Europe.

Shielding. Put heavy, dense, material between you and the source of the radiation. That is why paper works well. Hunker down in the middle of a library. Or a records center.

There are a series of alerts, curiously named mostly to prevent panic, that you should be aware of if you live near a reactor:

*Notification of Unusual Event*: a minor problem has occurred but no radiation has leaked or is expected to leak. We're just notifying you because the law says so and we want to scare you. But no action on your part is necessary.

*Alert*: A small problem has occurred and small amounts of radiation have or may leak inside the facility. This won't affect you—we hope—and you don't have to do anything. Personally, I'd be bugging out. Because they are, in essence, telling you they've had a breach of containment. They wouldn't be telling you that unless absolutely necessary.

*Site Area Emergency*: They're a little vague on this one. Area sirens may sound. Listen to your radio or television for safety info. I'd be listening to the radio while leaving.

*General Emergency*: Radiation could be coming off the plant site. Sirens are sounding. Tune to radio/TV for information. I'd check the information first, before bugging. Because you might be better off hunkering down inside your house than going through a radiation cloud.

Measures to be taken in a nuclear emergency:

Keep windows closed in your house and car. Use re-circulating air.

If you are advised to stay in your house, turn of the air conditioner, ventilation fans, furnace and any other air intakes into the house. Go to the basement or other underground area.

If you have been exposed to nuclear radiation take off all clothing. Bag it and seal it. Don't ever wear it again. Safely dispose of as soon as possible. Take a thorough shower. You are literally washing radiation off you. Put fresh, unexposed clothing on. Any exposed food should be disposed off.

The bottom line is to get as far away as quickly and as far as possible if you can.

129

## Nuclear Weapons

Duck and cover. How many remember that?

A nuclear attack could be limited to a single explosion or a World War.

Let's focus on what you should do:

First, a nuclear war probably won't happen in a vacuum. Keep an eye on the news. Currently the situation between Israel and Iran, or North and South Korea, are the most likely flashpoint for a nuclear exchange. It is more likely there could be a small yield nuclear explosion by terrorists and the will probably be a 'dirty' bomb.

We have DEFCON levels, which are defense readiness conditions for the Armed Forces.

**DEFCON 5:** lowest state of readiness. Supposed to be the norm.

**DEFCON 4:** Increased intelligence watch and strengthened security measures. Above normal readiness, but no running around screaming in the streets yet.

**DEFCON 3**: Increase in force readiness. This is when alerts go out to military forces to up their alert status. The Air Force is on 15 minutes notice to mobilize. Still no running around screaming but take some deep breaths.

**DEFCON 2:** The next step will be nuclear war. All military units are ready to engage in six hours. Start screaming.

**DEFCON 1:** Nuclear war is imminent. The code name for this is Cocked Pistol, which gives you an idea.

We've never gone to DEFCON 1. Publicly, we've gone to DEFCON 2 once, during the Cuban Missile Crisis. On 9-11, we went to DEFCON 3.

One sign that a nuke has gone off somewhere is the EMP effect. If all electronic devices suddenly fail, assume a nuclear bomb has been detonated high in the atmosphere and expect more to be coming.

If a nuke goes off, seek shelter immediately. The first sign of an explosion will be a flash, which travels at the speed of light. Behind the flash comes the shock wave, so you will have some moments to react. Do not look in the direction of the blast. If outdoors, seek a depressed area, exposing as little of your skin as possible. If indoors, get away from windows and fight the temptation to look to see what the bright light was about—the imploding window will likely kill you with lacerations. If you survive the initial blast, you have to take the correct steps to stay alive.

Most people who survive initially, will want to flee. However, this is the exact wrong thing to do. You are exposing yourself to fallout by fleeing. The blast has thrown a large amount of irradiated debris into the air. This fallout will be coming down. You don't want it to come down on you. Your goal is to place the most protection between you and the fallout and radiation. Ideally be underground.

Fallout tapers off relatively quickly. After an hour it's down about 50%. After a day it can be down to only 20%. So these first hours are critical.

After that, the issue is whether this has been a large-scale attack or a local event. If a local event, wait for responders. If a large-scale event, time to bug out.

*Infectious Diseases and Biological and Chemical Weapons and Accidents*

A pandemic will most likely consist of a virus. Viruses are tiny organisms, 100 times smaller than a single bacteria cell. They are an infective agent that typically consists of a nucleic acid molecule in a protein coat that is able to multiply only within the living cells of a host. Thus, by itself, the virus is not alive. It needs a host. When a virus infects a host, it invades the cells and take them over in order to carry out its own life process of multiplication and growth.

131

An infected cell produces viral particles instead of doing its normal functions. When a virus infects a host, it invades the cells and take them over in order to carry out its own life process of multiplication and growth. An infected cell produces viral particles instead of doing its normal functions.

Anthrax is the most likely agent to be used. It is pretty much 100% deadly when it enters a person's lungs. A minimum fatal dose is one spore and the problem is the symptoms don't show up for days. However, the spores are highly static and tend to clump together and with dust and dirt, making them too big to actually get into the lungs. Thus a package containing anthrax would be very dangerous to the person opening it, or an anthrax bomb deadly for those directly exposed to it, but beyond that immediate circle, others could quickly clear the area and be safe, because it has a very low rate of secondary uptake. This means once it's on the ground, it tends to stay there. So if you are in an area where anthrax is released, go to a sealed room and wait it out. Of more concern is smallpox, because it spreads more easily and is more persistent, although its lethality rate is lower. The problem is that you must quarantine people who are exposed because symptoms might not appear for several weeks.

### What are the Six Stages of a pandemic?

The World Health Organization has a Six Stage influenza program, plus two Periods:

**Stage 1** No animal influenza virus circulating among animals have been reported to cause infection in humans.

**Stage 2** An animal influenza virus circulating in domesticated or wild animals is known to have caused infection in humans and is therefore considered a specific potential pandemic threat.

**Stage 3** An animal or human-animal influenza reassortant virus has caused sporadic cases or small clusters of disease in people, but has not resulted in human-to-human transmission sufficient to sustain community-level outbreaks.

**Stage 4** Human-to-human transmission of an animal or human-animal influenza reassortant virus able to sustain community-level outbreaks has been verified.

**According to the WHO, if an influenza pandemic were to emerge today, we could expect:**

As people today are highly internationally mobile, the pandemic virus would spread rapidly around the world.

Vaccines, antiviral agents, and antibiotics to treat secondary infections would quickly be in short supply.

Several months would be needed before any vaccine became available. This is because some pandemic viruses are new ones.

Medical facilities would be overwhelmed.

There would be sudden and potentially considerable shortages of personnel to provide vital community services as the illness became widespread.

**Stage 5** The same identified virus has caused sustained community level outbreaks in two or more countries in one WHO region.

**Phase 6** In addition to the criteria defined in Phase 5, the same virus has caused sustained community level outbreaks in at least one other country in another

WHO region.

**LOST PEAK PERIOD** Levels of pandemic influenza in most countries with adequate surveillance have dropped below peak levels.

**POST PANDEMIC PERIOD** Levels of influenza activity have returned to the levels seen for seasonal influenza in most countries with adequate surveillance.

*What To Do?*

Depending on where you live and how much you travel will determine what your chances of getting infected. If you live in an urban setting, the chances are higher. Whether it's a pandemic or just the flu, here are basic steps to take:

Cover your nose and mouth with a tissue when you cough or sneeze. Throw it away after use.

Use a mask if you become aware that people are getting sick. Actually, it might look odd seeing those people in airports wearing a mask, but it's a good idea. Better to look a bit foolish than catch something that will make you sick and might possibly kill you.

Wash your hands with soap and water. Use disinfection.

Stay away from the sick people.

Stay away from crowds.

If it's a true pandemic, it's not likely that a hospital is a place to go as it will quickly become overwhelmed with the sick and dying.

The bottom line is to stay aware and isolate yourself and your team as quickly as possible.

If you are at home when there is a chemical/biological attack or accident, shut all air intake into the house: windows, doors, garage. Turn off your heating/air conditioning. You do not want air circulating inside the house or coming in from outside. Choose the room that has the least windows and doors. Run tape along any windows where there are seams. Cover the windows with polyethylene sheeting.

You should have one room in the house designated as the safe room to survive the initial stages of a nuclear, chemical or biological incident. When you have all team members and supplies in the room, finish sealing it by taping around the door, paying particular attention to the gap between the bottom of the door and the floor. You can use a wet towel and then tape it over. Look for any air vents (either in or out) and seal those with sheeting.

# Specific Natural Disasters

### Tornado

Tornados strike with little warning. If an alarm or alert has been sounded, even if you don't see one, assume it's there. Seek shelter. NOW!

Underground is always best for a shelter. Those areas that are prone to tornadoes have designated shelters. If your house is in a tornado area, you should have a room, a neighbor's house with a room, or a shelter already decided upon.

If a shelter is not available, go to the basement of a building. Stay away from windows and glass. Cover yourself with a mattress, cushions, blankets or a sleeping bag. Look around you for objects that could be blown over and don't be in their path if they fall.

If stuck in a building with no basement, go the lowest floor and the smallest room near the center of the house. Or under a stairwell or in an interior hallway with no windows.

Bathrooms are good because you have pipes in the wall which help strengthen them and you can lie in the bathtub. Lie on the ground, face down, and cover your head with your hands and arms. If you have a strong table, take cover under that. Cover yourself with cushions, blankets or a mattress.

Stay in your safe place until well after the danger has passed. Have your G&G bag with you with your crank radio so you can check in to the National Weather Service.

When you do leave your shelter, be careful. Avoid power lines and water that might be touched by power lines. Stay clear of buildings as they still might collapse. Avoid using open flame as it's likely there are gas leaks.

### Hurricane

Evacuate.

Board and tape windows. Plywood is best for covering window. For taping, use alligator tape, not duct tape. Masking tape is not useful.

Fasten your roof down to the house with tie down straps. Really long ones. You need to have these on hand *before* the hurricane is coming.

Turn off gas and/or propane.

clear away debris that can be picked up and smash into the house and windows.

Secure all outdoor furniture. If you have a pool, put the furniture into the water.

Make sure your garage doors are closed.

Looking at the deaths from Hurricane Sandy, over half of them were from falling trees/limbs. Make sure the trees around your house are properly trimmed and if old and unstable, pay to have them removed. It's worth your life and your family's lives.

As the storm approaches, turn your freezer and refrigerator to their coldest settings.

Pack any coolers with as much ice as possible. Use them first instead of opening the refrigerator door. If you grew up like I did, your dad was always yelling at your for opening the frig door anyway.

Fill bathtubs with water.

Make sure all vehicles are topped off.

Know where the closest shelter is for you and for your pets.

If you have to evacuate leave a note saying where you are going.

Unplug everything before leaving.

Turn off electricity, gas and water.

After the hurricane passes, beware of flooding.

Use flashlights or chem lights, never candles.

Do not use tap water after the storm until you are sure it isn't contaminated.

EVACUATE.

If you did not evacuate and it strikes, then you are in tornado mode.

**Heat Wave and Drought**

Keep your air-conditioning at a livable level. However, if there is a power outage or you don't have air-conditioning there are things to keep in mind. Lower floors are always cooler as heat rises. Close shades and lower blinds. Go somewhere that does have air conditioning such as a mall or theater.

Drink sufficient water but don't overdo it. During heat waves and also athletic events, there is the danger of *over-hydration*. This is a potentially fatal condition. Not long ago a student in Ranger School died from this. You drink too much water for your kidneys to process. It's not just the amount, but how quickly you drink the water.

Drinking too much water increases the amount of water in your blood. This dilutes the electrolytes, especially sodium. Sodium is critical in balancing the fluid inside and outside of cells. When there is an imbalance from over-hydration, sodium moves inside the cells, causing them to swell. This is particularly dangerous to your brain cells.

A dangerous thing about hyponatremia (what this is called) is that it can be confused with dehydration and people can force the victim to drink more water. Extreme sports athletes are at risk for this, as well people during a heat wave.

Without access to special medications, primary treatment for this to stop the water intake. If symptoms are not extreme, try to balance out the sodium with a sports that contains sodium.

Eat lighter meals during a heat wave so the body doesn't have work as hard digesting, producing more internal heat. Keep your skin covered. If outdoors, wear a hat to protect from sunlight. Wear lighter colors to reflect sunlight.

Use fans in your house to promote circulation of air. In the evening at night, open windows to let in cooler air, then close them in the morning along with blinds and shades.

Turn off extra sources of heat such as lights and appliances. Don't use the stove or oven.

Avoid alcohol and caffeine as they are diuretics and dehydrate you.

Recognize heat-related illness symptoms. Covered under first aid earlier in this manual.

Remember your pets. They also suffer in a heat wave. Put them in the shower. Give them a cool, wet towel to lie on. Make sure they have plenty of water to drink.

Heat waves contribute to drought.

Use rain barrels and other ways of collecting rain water. The typical roof produces 500 gallons of run off from just one inch of rain! Typically the water is considered non-potable, but it can be used for a variety of uses, and can be filtered in an emergency.

Make sure the dishwasher and clothes washer are full before using.

Don't leave water running on a faucet. Take shorter showers.

| Water Usage | |
| --- | --- |
| Dishwasher | 8 to 12 gallons per load |
| Clothes washer | 50 gallons per load |
| Shower | 3 to 5 gallons per minute |
| Running faucet | 2 to 3 gallons per minute |

Remember that drought can lead to . . .

**Wild Fire**

The wind throws embers one mile or more ahead of the flames. These embers start new fires. A fast wild fire has an intense wall of heat in front of it. Even if the flames haven't arrived, it will combust the most flammable material.

As the main fire approaches your house, strong winds blow embers everywhere possible – under decks, against wood fences, into woodpiles, and through open doors and windows. Embers blown onto the roof can come to rest in piles of dry leaves.

In some places the air is so smoky that you can't see more than 10 feet.

Close to where the fire is burning most intensely, the air is far too hot to breathe.

The rising smoke and ash create winds on the ground cause all the fires to burn even more intensely.

Fires like this occur every year. Wild fires don't just happen in the summer; in many areas fires can happen year round. When it is dry and windy be watchful and be prepared to take action to protect your family and property.

*To prepare your home if you live in an area prone to wildfires, here is a list of things to do:*

Keep your roof and gutters free of leaves.

Store firewood at least 30 feet away from structures. The nice pile up against the side of your house is called fuel for a wildfire.

Your outdoor furniture should be made of noncombustible materials.

Clear the area around your house of other combustible material such as leaves, bark, pine needles and underbrush. Especially trim grass and brush around your propane tank. Optimally you want a hundred foot barrier of no trees, shrubs or bushes around your house.

When building walls, barriers, gates, landscaping, etc use noncombustible materials.

When evacuating a wildfire, you should leave as soon as you receive notice. Considering there is a chance your house might not be there for you to come back to, besides your G&G bag, also take that fireproof container with all your key documents in it. And your pets. Beyond that, forget about it. Just like below, when discussing a tsunami, people are more important than any keepsake. And wild fires move fast!

While evacuating, make sure you have enough gas. This goes back to always keeping your tank at least half full and having at least a five gallon spare can that you can grab to take with you.

Leave any gates open for firefighters and others.

Drive with headlights on. If it's smoky, close all windows, and recirculate air inside the vehicle.

If you get trapped, park in an area that is clear of vegetation (parking lot, gravel area, dirt), close all windows and vents, cover yourself with a blanket or coat and lie on the floor. Car tires may burst from heat.

In an extreme situation, you have to consider whether you can stay in your house only if: your only escape route is blocked; smoke is so thick you can't travel; you don't have time to evacuate; or emergency personnel tell you to.

You cannot stay in your house if: you have wood siding or shingles; you're located in a narrow canyon or on a steep slope; you have a lot of vegetation close around the house. Find a neighbor with a better house.

If you do stay in a house, do the following: use a sprinkler or the sprinkler system to wet the yard. Wet the roof with a hose. Turn off all propane and gas. Close all windows and doors. Move fabric covered furniture away from large windows or sliding doors. Turn off everything that circulates air through the house. Close all interior doors.

On the opposite extreme from wild fires, there is . . .

### Blizzard

Like a hurricane, there is usually warning before a blizzard strikes. A blizzard is defined as a severe snowstorm with sustained winds over 35 miles per hour and lasting more than three hours.

Build your shelter. Get a fire going.

### Earthquake

If you're indoors, stay there.

Get under and hold onto a desk or table. Or stand against an interior wall.

Stay clear of exterior walls, glass, heavy furniture, fireplace and appliances.

Stay out of the kitchen.

If in an office building, stay away from exterior walls and glass.

Do not use elevators.

If you're outside, get into the open, clear of buildings, power lines, trees or anything else that can fall on you.

If you're driving, move the car out of traffic and stop. DO NOT park under bridges or overpasses. Get clear of trees, light posts and power lines. If you resume driving, watch out for road hazards, broken levels of roads, and downed power lines.

If you are in a mountainous area, be aware of the potential for landslides.

After an earthquake, watch out for fire hazards. Shut off valves for gas. If electrical wiring is damaged, turn off the main breaker.

If you are near the ocean be aware of . . .

### Tsunami

Again, you should be relatively well prepared based on what you've already done from this book. Here are specifics for a tsunami:

If you live in a tsunami zone, any earthquake should be cause for concern. Even one across the ocean.

If the water recedes suddenly, get out. Don't go pick up the flopping fish or you'll end up being one.

If animals start acting strangely, or running away, follow. Animals are often a good indicator that something in nature is abnormal. Often they are smarter than us. They don't grab a flashlight in a horror movie to go investigate that strange noise in the basement.

Evacuate when warned. Right away. Don't stop to gather personal items. Get your G&G and go.

Make sure you have a vehicle route and a walking route to higher ground. In the panic of evacuation, the vehicle route can turn into an obstacle.

*Bottom line, get to higher ground.* If you caught as it hits, climb a large tree, go up the stairs to the roof. Do not stop to watch the tsunami.

If you are caught in the water, grab onto something that floats. The real danger is being smashed against other objects. You also might get washed out to sea.

Do not return until officially notified. Sometimes tsunamis come in groups.

## Volcano

Leave immediately if ordered to evacuate. Keep tuned in on your radio for the latest updates.

Get to high ground. Lava follows the rule of gravity. Don't try to outrun it, try out-altitude it.

Avoid breathing poisonous gasses. Do not go to low ground as gasses accumulate there.

The gas flow from an eruption can expand at over 300 miles an hour.

Beware of roof collapse if a lot of ash is being deposited.

Never try to cross a lava flow even if it appears the surface has cooled and solidified.

Most people die in mudflows and flooding after an eruption. Thus, even though you are out of the immediate danger, be aware of these other dangers.

## Mud/Land Slide

Warning signs:

Periods of heavy rainfall or snow melt saturate the ground and cause instability in sloped areas. Areas prone to earthquakes, hurricanes, wildfires and other natural disasters are also prone to slides. Roads cut through hills and mountains are susceptible since the natural geography has been disturbed. Locations at the base of steep ridgelines, hills and mountains are in danger.

If you're in a building and notice cracks developing in the walls, that's a sign that trouble is coming. More signs:

If doors and windows begin to get jammed.

Utility lines start to break.

Fences, poles, and trees start to tilt.

Water starts accumulating in abnormal places.

The terrain starts to bulge or starts slanting at the base of the slope.

GET OUT.

If trapped in your home as its occurring, move to the highest floor.

### Dams

Get out of channels below the dams. Most people killed in a dam emergency are caught by the massive amount of water being channeled downstream and the debris carried with it.

If you have time before an evacuation prepare your home as noted earlier.

Avoid moving water. Even just half a foot of rushing water can take your feet out from under you. The odds are you won't drown: you'll get bashed to death as you are tumbled downstream.

### Flood

A flood WATCH means a flood is possible.

A flood WARNING means the flood is happening.

If you have time, move valuables in your house to the highest level before evacuating.

When evacuating, move to higher ground, away from water sources, such as rivers and lakes.

Never go around a barrier on a road during a flood. It's there for a reason. To keep you from being dumb.

If evacuating in your car, avoid standing water. Drive very, very slowly. Many people have lost their lives driving into a dip in the road and submerging their vehicle. If you live in a flood zone, prepare your car as I described for the boat/ferry.

Don't walk through moving water. Even very shallow water can knock you off your feet and sweep you into deeper water.

Flash floods kill a lot of people every year. Here are the keys:

Never drive through a flooded road or bridge.

Stay to high ground.

Keep track of weather information. Just because it's not raining where you are, doesn't mean it's not raining up-water.

Do not stay in a flooded car.

If the car is swept away or submerged, stay calm and wait for the vehicle to fill with water. The doors will not open before then (although you might try to get out the sunroof). Open the door, hold your breath, and swim for the surface. You will now be in the current. Point your feet downstream. Go over obstacles, never under. Strive to angle toward dry ground, but don't fight directly against the current.

If you are stuck above the flash flood, such as in a tree, stay in place and wait for rescue rather than risking the fast-moving water.

# STOCKPILE, SCAVENGE, SUSTAIN

These are the three stages of dealing with emergencies and natural disasters.

## Stockpile

You've already done this using *Prepare Now*. However, if there is an impending emergency or natural disaster, you still have some time to do more.

Stockpile up to mild level initially, then move on to moderate and then extreme.

## Scavenge

You will probably begin scavenging even while in the stockpile stage if the emergency or catastrophe is a high level moderate or extreme. If you can add to your supplies, do so. Legally.

The two variables are expected length of the emergency and type.

## Sustain

Sustainment occurs when it becomes clear things will not return to normal.

You are already in the stockpile stage. You've prepared your home, your ERP, your car, and your Grab-n-Go bags. So let's discuss Scavenge and Sustain.

# Scavenge

Consider this stage two ways. The most obvious is when you have to do the scavenging. But there is also the danger of those who try to scavenge you and your stockpile, since you are already prepared.

*Defense against scavenging*: Here are keys:

Be aware of your situation. What are current threats, growing threats and potential threats?

Avoid conflict if at all possible.

Are you armed? Are you willing to use your weapons?

Make your situation a hard target. Simple scavengers go for the easiest targets first. How many people know you have stockpiled supplies? This is not something you want to broadcast. If they know, do they know you are also prepared to defend your home?

Act decisively. This is something you should have done during your Area Study. How far are you willing to go to defend your home and when will you bug out? You will go even further to defend your ERP/base camp, because you wouldn't be in them if it wasn't a high moderate to extreme emergency.

Be prepared to retreat. You defend up to a point, but discretion is smarter than being overwhelmed. Part of bugging out of your home is when you know it is no longer defendable. In your ERP/base camp, you have designated

147

your Rally Point and kept your Grab-n-Go bag packed. In the face of overwhelming attack, retreat.

Your first choice is to scare scavengers off. Your second is to retreat. Your last option is to incapacitate scavengers. If you go to this mode it's all or nothing.

A sad reality of extreme situations is that the bad people will be more decisive and act more ruthlessly than the good people.

You want to be the alive people.

There is a line between scavenging and looting. That lines moves as the situation becomes more extreme. In a life and death situation, there is no line.

People will loot if given the opportunity. A power outage in an urban environment is one such opportunity. During this, your goal is stay secure. Looters are not looking for things they need to survive. They're simply criminals taking advantage of the situation.

The timeline on when people turn into scavenger depends, but during Hurricane Katrina, things deteriorated quickly after only 48 hours.

Scavengers take only what they need for survival. However, scavenging other people in a survival situation is criminal and unethical. You scavenge places, not people.

# Where to Scavenge

This is only limited by your imagination and location. As with every topic, there are so many variables, so there are no hard and fast rules.

A major consideration is to accept that if you are in scavenge mode, so are others. Less prepared people will actually go into those mode *before* you do. Thus, they will be more experienced. They will also be more desperate.

Be counter-intuitive. Don't go for the obvious.

Where to scavenge will be determined by what supplies you need in priority order. How much you scavenge depends on how desperate your situation is.

This is something you should have considered during your Area Study. Take a look at your map. What's in the area? Housing, factories, parks, businesses, hospitals, schools, etc.?

The following is a list of locations, along with what can be found there. Note that some places will yield supplies you might not expect to find there.

**Houses.** Make sure any home you scavenge isn't occupied. It's not worth fighting over. You'll search depending on your needs. Meds? Food? Clothing? Don't forget the attic, basement and garage. Garages can yield surprising results. Consider sustainment items such as seeds and gardening tools. Trash bags for waterproofing and carrying your supplies. Something that people will miss are water filters! A high end home might have very effective filters that you can rip out and use at your base camp. Coffee filters are also useful to clean water before having to boil it. View the house as you did when you were looking at your own house for survival. There is drinkable water in the same places—the water heater for example.

**Apartment buildings.** More bang to time than single houses as they hold multiple homes. Don't forget the parking garage where you can search . . .

**Cars and trucks.** If you are mobile in your own vehicle you can scavenge gas and parts. However, vehicles can yield other supplies such as food, weapons, and water. Check the glove compartment. Check the trunk. Tire iron? Emergency kit? An car jack that can used to get into other places? Check the engine. Do you need the wiring? Does the battery still have life? Could you use the battery to start a fire? Tires can be burned to make an emergency signal with black smoke. NEVER use gas to start a fire. Mirrors can be used for signaling. Abandoned semi trucks can be full of whatever!

**ATV and Off-Road shop.** ATVs are a better form of transportation than cars in severe emergencies. Remember, vehicles require . . .

**Gas stations.** The obvious goal here is gas, although getting it out of the ground tanks without power requires you have to have a pump (battery or hand powered) and a long enough siphon hose. There are easier ways to get gas.

**Automotive stores.** For vehicles parts.

**Food and grocery stores.** These will be first targets of scavengers and will quickly be picked clean. Don't forget to check in the back, where the restock is. You might consider *avoiding* these places in the early stages of an extreme emergency. After all, you have your own stockpile. Perhaps bypass the stores and go to the . . .

**Distribution Center**. During your Area Study, did you find local and regional distribution centers for stores? These will be full of supplies and not initially be on most people's scavenging radar as they go for the low hanging fruit first. Don't forget to check the semi-trailers parked outside that might not have been unloaded or recently loaded.

**Restaurants.** Food, but also check for knives, pots and pans.

**Bars.** You really don't need alcohol, but check for bottled water. Weapons hidden under and behind the bar.

**Schools (including colleges and community colleges)**. First aid kits. Tools in the maintenance room. Does it have a shop class?

**Hospitals.** What are you priorities medically? Again, though, these will be among the first targets for scavengers. Also, they will be a place people will congregate. Depending on the threat, it might also harbor the threat, such as a pandemic.

**Pharmacies.** Initially people will go for the drugs. There are other items that might be overlooked. Ace wraps are very useful for a variety of things. Bandages. While most people think of hospitals and pharmacies first for medical supplies, consider these . . .

**Veterinarians and animal hospitals.** These are stocked with medical supplies, including medications

**Nursing homes.** Ditto.

**Storage units.** It's certain some people have put their emergency stash in a locked storage unit. In addition, there are all sorts of supplies to be found, concentrated in one place.

**Office buildings.** Often they will have first aid kits and some emergency gear in them. Consider what kind of business it was. What will be there? Check desk drawers.

**Police stations.** Weapons. Tools. Emergency kits. Radios.

**Fire stations.** First aid kits, emergency tools, radios. A pump truck could hold hundreds of gallons of water. Don't assume its potable.

**Military posts and National Guard Armories.** If abandoned, they might contain weapons and other equipment. However, to get to a level where you're scavenging, the National Guard and military were most likely already called out and deployed.

**Animal Control Centers.** Guess where you can find traps?

**Dumpsters.** One man's trash is another man's treasure. They can also be shelters.

**Dumps.** You never know.

**Train stations.** Vending machines, restaurants. Check the bathrooms. The lockers.

**Trains.** Check the luggage.

**Airports.** There are supplies inside an airport and restaurants and stores. Also, think of the parking lots, rich with all those vehicles. And gas in those cars.

**Aircraft.** Check the galley. The luggage.

**Marinas.** Check not only the marina, but abandoned boats. A boat can be an excellent base camp, depending on the threat, where you are, and if you know what you're doing.

**Farms**. Look not only at the house and the barn, but what's being grown. Could it be a source of sustainable food?

**Libraries and bookstores**. This is a place that almost all scavengers will bypass or ignore, but is the most important if you are in scavenge mode. Because it is possible you will transition from scavenge mode into sustain mode, rather than recovery. Books are knowledge. Knowledge is power. You have this book. Get others that are on topics you need and will need. Get books that will help you transition into sustainment. How to farm. How to make things.

# How to Scavenge

When on the move in an emergency or catastrophe, you should always be on the lookout for useful materials as needed. Don't hoard, but complement what you already have. Also, save your stockpile of prepared material as much as possible by using scavenged supplies.

If you are in your home, ERP or base camp and need supplies, you must plan a scavenging expedition. This not something to be done lightly. If you are in scavenge mode, so are others. And you are all looking for the same supplies.

That's the first planning consideration. What are the priorities of supplies needed? You don't simply list everything you need. You prioritize. People can only carry so much, but you might also have your scavenging time cut short by the presence of others.

After you have determined the scavenging objective (location and priorities of supplies), the first step is to send a scout. The scout should have optics and a way to communicate back. It is optimal to put 24 hours of surveillance on any target. The scout must have a communication schedule to strictly follow and a time limit to return. If either of those two pass, you must consider the scout compromised, along with your location.

The scout should check the objective for ingress and egress. Dangers. Special equipment that will be needed, such as bolt cutters. Whether the objective is damaged and dangerous structurally.

Once the scout reports back, it's time to put together the expedition. Never send someone alone. Always work in at least buddy teams. Someone is designated as the leader. Factors include how much is needed and how much can be carried. Plan security on the move and at the objective. Everyone should carry:

A backpack. As many empty bags as they can carry when full. Also remember, you can scavenge a location and then spend time moving material out and caching it nearby where other scavengers wouldn't look. Then go back for it.

Everyone should have gloves, multitool, flashlight, and weapon. The expedition should have at least one crowbar. If you are scavenging gas, you need a siphon and containers.

The scavenging party must have a Rally Point where they will regroup if attacked or forced to disperse while on the expedition. This Rally Point is *not* simply going back to the home/ERP/camp. In fact, it should be in a direction that will not lead others to the home/ERP/camp.

If going into a large building, you must have a way to mark your way back out. Glow sticks, spray paint, markers. Remember, any mark you leave tells other you exist and were there.

Scavenging is only limited by your imagination, your resources, your environment and the type of emergency/catastrophe.

# CONGRATULATIONS

Since you made it this far because you were well-prepared and knowledgeable, you are a true survivor.

If it was a mild or low end moderate emremgency, such as a power outage for several days, you expect things to return to normal eventually. The same with a hurricane you evacuated from. As you now know, the possibilities are endless. It might have been a personal extreme emergency or a localized emergency and now outside help is here to help in recovery. Here's what to do:

If you've been injured or sick, seek medical help.

Contact your loved ones. Let them know you're okay and make sure they are too.

Check your surroundings and make sure it really is safe.

Help out others who need assistance.

Contact your insurance company. Find out what it needs. Get a damage assessment.

Before you start cleaning up, make sure its safe to do so. Is your home stable? Is it safe to enter? You might have to get help.

Be careful of scams. Sad to say, there are those who prey on those who've just gone through trauma.

# SUSTAIN AND THRIVE

If things have not recovered to pre-emergency conditions, and it doesn't look like they will in the foreseeable future, you are into Sustain. While water and food and medicine and ammunition, etcetera are essential getting to this phase, there is a point at which things will stabilize and you will look past the present and simple survival to the future.

The future must be more than just survival. We want mankind to *thrive* when we start over.

The most important things you will need is knowledge and experience. That comes in two forms. Books and people. This is why the last place list listed in where to scavenge is libraries/bookstores.

The reality is that we have become very ignorant of the everyday processes of civilization that we take for granted. We're used to going to the store to get food, turning on the tap, having our cell phone work with no clue exactly how it was made or how it works.

If you're at this point of Sustain, that veneer has been stripped away. Technology has mostly, if not completely, failed.

You need not only the base knowledge, but also how to use the knowledge. You need the seeds of civilization. With the proper seeds, you can leapfrog history and accelerate recovery. A rebooted civilization will not look like what we have now. It will be a curious patchwork.

I use the word Sustain because before we move forward, we need to have achieved a sustainable level of living. The keys to a sustainable level are:

Sufficient food and water to support the community.

Clothes and shelter.

Medicine.

Building materials, sources of energy.

There is a flow by which we can regain much of what was lost. It's beyond the scope of this book to cover it, along with the information needed. Here is how you go about it as you have now passed the threshold of sustainment:

*Have adequate supplies.* You have a renewable source of water. Your gardening, hunting and gathering is sufficient that food is not an emergency concern. You have adequate medical supplies. Much of your supplies were gathered by scavenging.

*Pick a location.* You might stay in your ERP/base camp location. Or it might be wise to relocate to a better spot. With better resources. Better defenses. This depends on too many factors for us to pre-determine.

*Gather people.* People bring knowledge, skills, and physical and emotional support. You need to build a community. You want people with these skills:

Medical

Law enforcement and military

Electrical

Leadership

Survival

Child care

Communications
Engineering
Weapons
Gardening
Those are basics. But there is a role for everyone.

*Gather knowledge.* When you gather people, you are gathering knowledge. But you want sustainable knowledge.

Physical books are the key. Thus we are back to the library and book store. Electronic books are nice, but they need power. There will most likely be a gap between the power going out and the power being restored that needs to be bridged.

Gather books on topics based on a priority of needs. Make sure they are safely stored.

They are your future and your children's' future!

# This book is full of practical advice. However, the most important tool in a survival situation is your will to survive!

# If you've gotten this far, you can go further!

# The Key Phrase to Remember: SURVIVAL

The most important tool for survival is having the right mindset. All the training, preparation, information, tools, etcetera, are useless without the will to survive. This will is birthed from having the right mindset.

Don't be intimidated. The will to survive is in every person. Luckily, for most of us, we haven't had to tap into it. But when you have to, *you will*. Human beings are amazingly adaptable. I've talked to many people who say: If it's that bad, I don't want to survive. But my experience says you'll react differently. And when you do, this book will have you ready.

Here are some tools to help you:

The word **_Survival_** provides you with the first letters of the keys you need.

**S** - Size up the situation, your surroundings, yourself, and your equipment.

**U** - Use All Your Senses & Undue Haste Makes Waste

**R** - Remember Where You Are

**V** - Vanquish Fear and Panic

**I** - Improvise

**V** - Value Living

**A** - Act Like the Natives

**L** - Live by Your Wits

## S: Size up the situation, your surroundings, yourself, and your equipment.

There are two ways to do this: one is in preparation and the other is in the actual situation. For preparation, you size up your potential situations by doing an Area Study, which will we go through in detail later in the book.

_Size up your situation:_ Focus on what exactly is the threat in order of priority? This might seem obvious, but consider the situation in Japan in 2011. The initial event was the earthquake. That, however, wasn't the primary threat. The resulting tsunami caused much more devastation. And following that, the problems at the nuclear plants presented immense issues that are still having an effect.

_Size up your surroundings:_ When in a situation, tune in to the environment. Wherever you are, you are part of a system. This is key to survival. You don't want to fight your environment; you want to work with it. There is a pattern to nature. In an urban environment there are also patterns. Make note of the patterns and also focus on any time the pattern is disturbed.

One thing that always struck me was that no matter where my A-Team went in the world, no matter how hard we tried to hide, no matter how far from civilization we were, the locals always knew we were there,. Because our presence was abnormal. They sensed it. We weren't part of the normal pattern. Do the same with your environment.

*Size up yourself:* Have you, or someone on your team, been hurt or wounded? Often, in the initial rush of a trauma, we miss potentially lethal injuries. We'll discuss emergency first aid later, but you must take the time to assess everyone's physical condition. For example, with gun shot wounds, the exit wound can often be more dangerous than the entrance wound, but often people don't look for it.

Keep yourself healthy. Dehydration, which we'll cover under water, is a major problem that can easily be avoided. Notice how this is emphasized in *The Hunger Games*. The first piece of advice the mentor gives to the two candidates from his district is to find water. We can survive quite a while without food, but water is critical. Cold and wet are also enemies that you have to monitor and deal with.

*Size up your equipment:* What do you have? What can you get? What condition is your equipment in? This will be covered in more detail later on, but some situations might require field expediency. What do you have that is necessary and what can you do without? People have been killed in natural disasters by trying to carry too much stuff with them. During the tsunami in Japan many people died while they tried to pick up what they felt were irreplaceable items. Some people even went back to their houses after initially evacuating and died. The most important things are people, not memorabilia or jewels or money.

Nothing is more valuable than life.

## U - Use All Your Senses, Undue Haste Makes Waste

*Use all your senses.* A key trait, which mystifies many people, is called 6th sense. Great point men in the army are valued for this trait. They'll be leading a patrol along a trail and suddenly stop. Something has alerted them, but they can't pinpoint it right away. We all have 6th sense, but many of us don't pay attention to it. 6th sense is one or more of your other 5 senses picking up something real and alerting your subconscious. You actually saw or smelled or felt something, but didn't consciously register it. Trust that feeling. Focus and shift whatever it is to your conscious mind. Listen, smell, taste, touch, see. All are critical.

*Undue haste makes waste:* Unless you are in imminent danger, slow down and think things through. Panic is a killer. If you don't think and plan, you could do the wrong thing and in some cases cause a "no do-over" action, which is usually fatal. Don't take an action or move just for the sake of doing something. Every action and movement must have a purpose.

The good news is that once you finish this book and have done the checklists you will be so much more ready and have anticipated many potential problems and are prepared for them.

### R - Remember Where You Are

Know your location at all times. Also, know where the people on your team are. Stay oriented. Often you can use significant terrain features for that, whether it be a coastline, a mountain range, a river. They can also give you boundaries.

We'll go over traditional map reading later in this book because we have become overly reliant on GPS. We'll discuss maps, how to get them for free, how to use them, and field expedient direction finding techniques. It's a lot easier than you think it is.

Make sure everyone in the group is oriented. Make sure you know who has the map and compass. The map is inside a waterproof case. The map and compass are tied off to your body with a 'dummy' cord. Never rely on others to know where you're located. If you are moving, make note of key terrain features and water sources. Remember, water sources are where game congregates and usually have fish in them, so they are also food sources.

During my training at the International Mountain Climbing School, an experienced mountaineer told us a key to his surviving situations where others had perished: while going up the mountain, he repeatedly looked *back*. He wanted to see what it would look like when he was coming down the mountain. More people get lost and killed coming down the mountain than going up. We'll cover emergency rally points later, but once your team/family goes there on a visit, it will be easy for them to find it in an emergency.

## V - Vanquish Fear and Panic

Courage is acting in the face of fear. We are all capable of being heroes. And it's easier to be a here when you're prepared, which you will be.

Don't let your imagination run too far in a fatalistic direction, much like the one soldier in *Aliens* who kept screaming "We're all going to die." You don't want someone like that on your team.

Think about times in your life when you were in a crisis. How did you react? How did those people you want on your team react in a crisis? How someone reacts in a crisis gives you a very good idea of someone's core personality type in a survival situation.

Panic and fear also drain your energy. You're not focused on what needs to be done; you're focused on what could possibly go wrong. One way to help lower fear and panic is to be prepared, have a plan, and practice aspects of survival training so you build your confidence.

Which you're doing right now, by reading this book.

### I - Improvise

Look at the things around you with a different mindset in a survival situation. What might have one particular use in civilization can have a very different use in a survival situation.

No matter how well prepared you are, in an extended emergency, some of your gear will wear out. How can you use other objects around you? We'll cover some readily available objects and how they can be turned into other useful tools.

### V - Value Living

This harkens back to the opening of this book. The will to survive. You have it; tap into it.

Two men with similar wounds. One lived and one died. What was the difference? The one who lived wanted to with every atom of his being. The one who died succumbed to his fear and pain. He didn't value his life enough.

We tend to be creatures of comfort. Civilization has advanced to the point where few people have the day to day survival skills that many people had just a few generations ago. We buy our food prepared and pre-packaged. Our water comes from a tap. Electricity is taken as a given, rather than a precarious luxury. However, don't let that make you think you can't handle a survival situation.

One thing I have seen is that when people value living, they adapt surprisingly quickly. Most of our life consists of habits. When we are forced to change our habits, we rapidly adopt new ones.

No matter how hard it gets, never quit.

### A - Act Like the Natives

If you are out of your natural environment, then observe those around you, both human and animal. Those that are native to the area have adapted to it. What do they eat? Where do they get their food and water? Are there places they avoid? What are their customs and habits? Remember, even customs that seem very strange, often have a very practical root.

Watching animals is key. They also need water, food and shelter. Animals can also be an alert for the presence of other humans. And they can alert others to your presence.

If you are a stranger, gain rapport with the locals. In order to get respect, you have to show respect first.

## L - Live by Your Wits, But for Now, Learn Basic Skills

There are skills you need to practice now, actions you need to rehearse before having to use them in an emergency. I will highlight these skills as we go through the book. Again, preparation is the key to success, both in terms of equipment and training.

### Additional traits survivors have:

Above all a *determination to survive*. All else is secondary. Even if things look hopeless, you can't ever give up. Later in this book I'll give you examples where ordinary people who were thrust into extraordinary circumstances and did unbelievable things to survive. Things they never thought they were capable of.

You're capable of what is unimaginable to you right now.

In Special Forces we found a *sense of humor* could make the most difficult situation look a little brighter. In my team Standing Operating Procedures, under my commander's policy letter, the last thing listed was to "keep your sense of humor, you're going to need it." Laughter can be a pressure release. That's a big reason why I put it in this book. When we take ourselves too seriously, we lose track of the purpose of surviving.

As part of that, you also need to be able to *let it go*. Don't dwell on bad luck, past mistakes, or losses. Negative thinking drains energy. Look to the future. Deal with the present, prepare for the future and accept you can't change the past.

But you also don't control everything in the future either. You have to face it with a positive attitude but also accept that the *future is uncertain*. This entire book is based on that fact. It would be great if your current situation continues and you never face an emergency or survival situation or accident or disaster, but you have no guarantees. One symptom of disaster situations is that there will be considerable confusion and disinformation initially. Both because it won't be clear what's going on, but also factor in people spreading false information to further their own ends or sprouting from their fear and panic. You have to sort through it all and make the best possible decisions.

We're in this together.

In conclusion, you will find that the traits of the survivor are also the traits, in everyday, normal living, make a person successful. So you can use this book not only to prepare, but also to learn traits that will make your current environment more fruitful and positive.

# SURVIVAL

S  Size up the situation, your surroundings, yourself, and your equipment

U  Use All Your Senses & Undue Haste Makes Waste

R  Remember Where You Are

V  Vanquish Fear and Panic

I  Improvise

V  Value Living

A  Act Like the Natives

L  Live by Your Wits

# Books by Bob Mayer

## NON FICTION TITLES

*Who Dares Wins*
*Write It Forward*
*Novel Writer's Toolkit*
*How We Made Our First Million*
*The Writer's Conference Guide*

# SCIENCE FICTION TITLES

ATLANTIS
*Atlantis*
*Atlantis: Bermuda Triangle*
*Atlantis: Devil's Sea*
*Atlantis: Gate*
*Assault on Atlantis*
*Battle for Atlantis*

AREA 51
*Area 51*
*Area 51: The Reply*
*Area 51: The Mission*
*Area 51: The Sphinx*
*Area 51: The Grail*
*Area 51: Excalibur*
*Area 51: The Truth*
*Area 51: Nosferatu*
*Area 51: Legend*

NIGHTSTALKERS
*Nightstalkers*
*Nightstalkers: The Book of Truths*
*Nightstalkers: The Rift*

TIME PATROL
*Time Patrol*
*Time Patrol: Black Tuesday*
*Time Patrol: The Ides of March*
*Time Patrol: D-Day*
*Time Patrol: Independence Day*
*Time Patrol: Nine Eleven*

PSYCHIC WARRIOR
*Psychic Warrior*
*Psychic Warrior: Project Aura*

*The Rock*
*I, Judas The Fifth Gospel*

BOB MAYER

# THRILLERS

BRAND NEW FICTION
*The Fifth Floor*

THE CELLAR SERIES
*Bodyguard of Lies*
*Lost Girls*

PRESIDENTIAL SERIES
The Jefferson Allegiance
The Kennedy Endeavor

THE GREEN BERET SERIES
*Eyes of the Hammer*
*Dragon Sim-13*
*Synbat*
*Cut Out*
*Eternity Base*
*Z: The Final Countdown*

THE HORACE CHASE SERIES
*Chasing the Ghost*
*Chasing the Lost*
*Chasing the Son*

SHADOW WARRIORS
*The Line*
*The Gate*
*Omega Missile*
*Omega Sanction*
*Section Eight*

# HISTORICALS

DUTY, HONOR, COUNTRY
*West Point to Mexico*
*Mexico to Sumter*
*Sumter to Siloh*

# About Bob Mayer

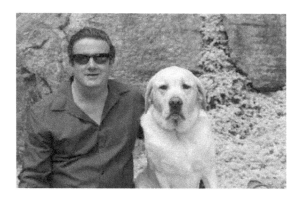

Bob Mayer is the grandfather of two future leaders of the Resistance Against the Machines, a NY Times Bestselling author, graduate of West Point, former Green Beret (including commanding an A-Team) and the feeder of two Yellow Labs, most famously Cool Gus. He's had over 70 books published including the #1 series Area 51, Atlantis, Time Patrol and The Green Berets. Born in the Bronx, having traveled the world (usually not tourist spots), he now lives peacefully with his wife, and labs in an undisclosed location.
http://bobmayer.com

To contact Bob Mayer and give feedback, suggestions, or other comments about *Prepare Now Survive Later*, please email at surivival@coolgus.com